GutBuster 2

The high energy guide

Garry Egger
and
Rosemary Stanton

Cartoons by Sue Plater

For men with the (decreasing)
gut to give it a go!

ALLEN & UNWIN

First published 1995
Allen & Unwin Pty Ltd
9 Atchison Street, St Leonards, NSW 2065 Australia

National Library of Australia
Cataloguing-in-Publication entry:

Egger, Garry.
  Gutbuster 2: The high energy guide.

  ISBN 1 86373 900 9.

  1. Weight loss. 2. Self-care, Health. 3. Men—Health
and hygiene. I. Stanton, Rosemary. II. Title. III. Title:
Gutbuster two.

613.25081

Set in 11/14pt Souvenir by DOCUPRO, Sydney
Printed by Griffin Paperbacks, South Australia

10 9 8 7 6 5 4 3 2 1

Contents

I
Background

1 Why the high energy guide?

When we produced the *GutBuster Waist Loss Guide* for men in 1992, we believed that it was the first book of its kind. Until then, most *weight* control books were distinctly female-oriented, distinctly diet-oriented, distinctly ignorant of the physiological and scientific facts and thus—in most cases—distinctly wrong!

We concentrated on men because men *are* different. Now that may sound like a glib statement, but in terms of structure, function, storage and loss of body fat, it can't be overstated. Men not only lose fat much more easily than women (when they want to), but they also store it in different parts of the body. Men respond differently to dieting and exercise, they generally lack knowledge about food and exercise and have fewer psychological hang-ups about being fat. While we do not dispute that this latter difference may be due to unfair social pressures, many of the former reflect very real physiological and psychological differences between the sexes that are often clouded by dust in the battle for equality.

The GutBuster Program is different because it rejects many of the accepted axioms of weight loss that have arisen from the over-emphasis on fat as a female problem. The first of these is that overfatness is more common among women. Traditional measures of obesity, such as the height and weight measures that go into a Body Mass Index (BMI), show that there are three over*weight* men to every two overweight women. More importantly, waist-to-hip ratio, which measures fat stored around the middle, shows that there are almost twice as many over*fat* men as women.

We also reject the notion of weight as a measure of fat. Weight can reflect muscle, bone density, water, organs and even *how long you grow your hair!* For this reason we suggested that you throw away your scales and stop weighing yourself. Even the next best measure, Body Mass Index, which measures weight in kilograms divided by height squared, has limited value in men because it doesn't take into account the fact that muscle is twice as dense as fat. A stocky, muscular man such as a football player might be obese by this measure, but hardly carry 'an ounce of fat'. The BMI has been used as a stop gap in measuring overweight because we had nothing better. Now, with improved technology and better measures of what is important, it is time it was replaced—or at least downgraded in importance.

Measuring fat, not weight

The best and easiest way to measure fat and fat loss, for a man in particular, is a simple tape measure around the belly. The measure is simple—it is done level with the navel and should be checked weekly. You can measure around the waist and the hips (at the widest point) to get a waist-to-hip ratio, which should be below 0.9 for optimum health for men (or below 0.8 for women). But, more simply, a long-term goal should be to get your waistline (irrespective of height), to below 100 cm (90 cm for women). Anything above this magnifies health risks.

The GutBuster Program aims for a 1 per cent loss around the waist each week at least over the first five weeks, then around 1 per cent per fortnight after that. For a woman, the best measure of excess fat is still to be determined. In Chapter 3 we explain why it is likely to be different from that of a man. But, for the moment, we can at least say that abdominal fat is a good indication of risk—even if not of fat—for a woman as well as a man. That is why GutBusters is called a 'Waist Loss' and not a *weight* loss program and why we talk only of *fat*, not *weight*, reduction.

The GutBuster 'Waist Loss' Program also differs from other guides in that it is really not a set program.

GB high energy tip

Throw your scales away and never weigh yourself again. Weight reflects water, muscle, bone and a lot of things other than fat. Measure around the waist instead of weighing.

There's no diet and no formal routine of exercises to do in lots of 10s or 20s. Diets and exercise routines are programs that you 'go on' and then 'come off' at some stage and are therefore unlikely to provide a long-term solution. The GutBuster Program is based on the belief that any changes that are made to a man's lifestyle HAVE to be able to be maintained for a lifetime. For that reason they HAVE to be enjoyable. If they are not, and they are not maintained, the program is a failure. For that reason we insist that men DON'T give up drinking; DON'T diet; DON'T drastically alter their lifestyle. These changes can't be maintained. As an alternative we proposed the concept of 'trading off'—alcohol for exercise, fibre for fat etc.—a practice that is much easier to live with over a lifetime.

We also dismissed the concept of the 'beer gut'. The *beer* gut is a myth. Not only do many big men not drink (often because they think that's what caused their problem), but many heavy drinkers and alcoholics have no sign of a 'beer gut'. In fact, in a recent study of all research carried out on alcohol intake and obesity, no simple relationship was shown. Other research has shown that alcohol, like carbohydrate in foods, is usually burned up or 'oxidised' as energy rather than stored as fat. Fat in foods, on the other hand, is usually stored as fat rather than oxidised as energy (the reasons are explained later). Fatty foods and alcohol together may cause a 'beer gut', because alcohol slows the burning of fat even further. But it is the fat and not the alcohol that causes the 'beer belly'.

> *The beer gut is a myth. Not only do*
> *many big men not drink, but many*
> *heavy drinkers and alcoholics have*
> *no sign of a 'beer gut'.*

For this reason the GutBuster Program, unlike others, doesn't blacklist alcohol. In fact it encourages moderate consumption because, in line with the first commandment (see below), we know that most men won't stay off the grog for life. We have, however, provided some special guidelines for drinking, such as not eating chips, peanuts or fatty foods with alcohol and choosing low calorie (not necessarily low alcohol) drinks.

Fat research

Another major difference between GutBusters and other *weight* control programs is in its use of new

---

The GutBuster 10 commandments

1 Only make changes you can stick to for life.
2 Become a 'fat detective'—seek out fats then seek to avoid them.
3 Move—anywhere, any time.
4 Trade off your indulgences.
5 Change WHAT and HOW you eat, not HOW MUCH.
6 Don't drink anything you can eat whole (e.g. eat fruit rather than drinking fruit juice).
7 Watch yourself—observe, monitor, record, reward.
8 See only 'opportunities' not 'inconveniences'.
9 'Stalk' your habits as the first stage of changing them.
10 'Shock' to 'unblock'—to get through plateaus and downers.

physiological research on fat and fat loss. In the 1980s, there was tremendous growth in exercise science. But it can take around ten years for information from scientists' laboratories to filter through to those for whom it matters. At the start of the 1990s, there was about as much biological and physiological information on fat in the scientific literature as there was on muscle in the late 1970s. Recently, this has begun to change with a flood of new research findings altering the basis of traditional weight control programs. Diets, for example, are now considered to be old hat or, even worse, counter-productive for fat loss over the long term. More emphasis is now placed on metabolism and modifying metabolic rate, one of the key aims of most good fat loss programs these days.

We introduced some new and novel ways of modifying metabolic rate in the first GutBuster Program, such as eating spicy food, drinking caffeine, not using doonas on the bed etc. Some of these have now become more established in the scientific literature. There have also been other major developments in health with implications for effective fat loss and high-level wellness. For example, a better understanding of food in fat loss (Chapters 5–8), more specific exercise prescription for fatness in contrast to fitness (Chapters 9–11), a finer appreciation of the differences in response between men and women (Chapter 3) and new evidence on men's lifestyle patterns that has implications for health programming (Chapter 2). In this program we also look again at behaviour change (Chapter 12) and motivation (Chapters 13–14) and examine the importance of stress (Chapters 15 and 16)

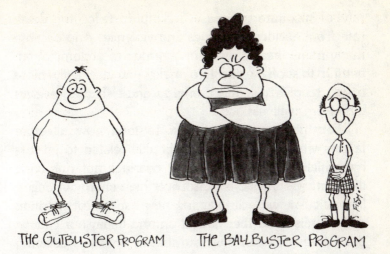

THE GUTBUSTER PROGRAM   THE BALLBUSTER PROGRAM

and other health risks associated with male fatness (chapters 17–18).

From waist loss to wellness

Perhaps one of the most important features of the GutBuster Program is that, although it emphasises fat (particularly around the middle), it is just as much about health and regaining control over one's life, as it is about reducing the 'garage over the tool shed'. Men traditionally have had difficulty discussing this with their doctors—or other men. Simply put, it's a bit 'wussey' to show an interest in your health if you're one of those who doesn't eat quiche. On the other hand, it is difficult to hide an abdominal enhancement. And yet men need to take an interest in their health. They die six years younger than women on average; they suffer twice the rate of heart disease, one-and-a-half times the rate of respiratory disease and up to twice the death rate from accidents, injuries and violence. And because many men's health problems are due to abdominal fat, getting this off is likely to make you decidedly more frisky, to give you more energy and a higher level of long-term wellness.

For this reason, we need to look now at other factors which may not seem directly related to fat loss but which can have important bearings not only over the portly poundage but also over high-energy wellness. In particular, we will examine new aspects of nutrition and exercise and the motivation and behaviour change procedures that can maintain these, as well as covering aspects of stress and how to control this, and even how to recognise and prevent the major diseases associated with fatness and middle age.

2 From fitness to fatness, or from caveman to computerman

In Shakespeare's seven ages of man (from *As You Like It*), he describes mid-life as:

> In fair round belly, with good capon lin'd,
> With eyes severe, and beard of formal cut,
> Full of wise saws and modern instances,
> And so he plays his part:

On the back of a toilet door (where most good modern philosophy is often written), it's explained like this:

> When I was what I was, I always wanted to be what I am now. But now that I am what I am, I wish I was what I was before I became what I wanted to be. (Anon.)

Many strange things can happen to men when they hit mid-life (and, let's face it, this can be at only 35–40 years of age). As many of these are unconscious, men are often not aware of them and most are more obvious from the outside than from the inside. It's a time when

11

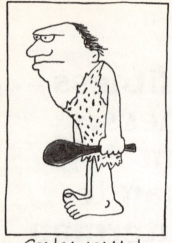

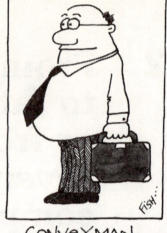

CONCAVEMAN   CONVEXMAN

some men leave a perfectly good family to fiddle in the dalliances of an almost lost youth—young women, flashy sports cars, bald heads, expanding middles.

But it is also a time when many physiological changes occur. The forty-something man is likely to wake up one morning and find that where bits were once hard, they're now soft, and where bits were once soft, they're now hard! Perhaps, unexpectedly, this softness is not only in the downstairs department. In particular, more softness begins to accumulate around the middle. It might not be noticeable at first, but it can grow almost imperceptibly to throw shade on parts thereunder. Lo and behold, before you know it, you've become a Pauncho Gonzales.

Why does it happen in the middle years? You may not seem to be eating or drinking any more and you probably haven't noticed a big change in the amount

---

GB High Energy Tip

Measure your waist (at the navel) regularly and aim to get it below 100 cm. This is the waist size (irrespective of height) above which health risks increase.

---

of exercise that you're doing. So something else is going on. What is it?

Put simply, your body is telling you that you are no longer a young buck. It does this mainly by slowing you down. Metabolic rate, or the rate at which your body burns energy, remains relatively stable in men until about the age of 40. After that, it tends to drop off in a linear fashion—probably by about 2–3 per cent per decade. That may not sound like much, but as about 70 per cent of the total energy that the body uses comes from your metabolism (that is, the energy required just to keep you alive), then 2–3 per cent of that can be quite significant. It can mean an extra kilogram of flab every six months!

Why around the middle ?

The males of the species *Homo sapiens* over the millennia were once the more active hunters of the tribe. Humanoids have evolved with males expending a lot of energy over brief periods to secure food. Females, on the other hand, expended much of their energy in rearing new additions to the species. The energy expenditure needed to produce breast milk is high and is one of the reasons why lactating mothers usually lose excess body fat acquired during pregnancy.

Historically, men needed an energy reserve that was

readily accessible when times got tough. There had to be food on the table (or maybe rock). It may have taken a day or two to catch animals for food and it may have been many days before more food was caught. Fat, the most efficient store of energy reserve, was (and still is) pocketed away in little sacks around the waist in men to allow for these times of need. Nature, in her wisdom, provided men with a rucksack full of sandwiches in case they were caught short!

Women, on the other hand, needed resilient fat that could help them survive the nine months of pregnancy and the high energy needs of breastfeeding to ensure the survival of the species. They store this in more resistant fat cells that tend to be situated around the hips and buttocks. Hence, you'll notice the typical apple or 'android' shape of those men who have become fat after adolescence, and the more pear or 'gynoid' shape of the typical woman. An 'ovoid' shape, with more overall fat (like the fruit box that the apple and pear come in), is common in the genetically obese.

In young boys and young men, belly fat is readily burned up, not just by the energy needed to catch wild animals, but by a high metabolic rate—the 'fire within'—which, like a gas heater pilot light, is the energy required for muscle growth and system maintenance. After adolescence, men stop growing and, as they get longer in the tooth, they tend to slow down a little. In times gone by, this would mean that they would be less efficient than their younger competition at running down their next meal. So the body helps out by providing a little more protection for survival. Energy use slows down through a decrease in metabolism—we

THE 3 FRUIT SHAPES OF MAN

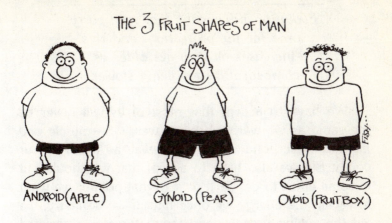

ANDROID (APPLE)   GYNOID (PEAR)   OVOID (FRUIT BOX)

no longer need energy to grow—and so fat is stored a little more easily around the middle, providing that extra reserve as a protection against leaner times. For this reason most middle-aged men—even the fit ones—carry a little extra fat around the middle which is much harder to lose than when they were younger.

Fat in evolution

It seems, then, that men carry some fat for protection, and this increases as they get older as compensation for being slower. Unfortunately, evolution has not catered for the excesses that exist in the twentieth century. Although it may be reasonable to expect an older man to carry a little bit extra around the middle as a kind of security blanket, the excess abdominal fat that is now characteristic of almost half of Australian men is known to be extremely dangerous.

> *Evolution has meant that men carry*
> *some fat for protection, and this*
> *increases as they get older as*
> *compensation for being slower.*

We have to accept that most of us will never be the same as we were when we were 18—muscle and fat fails to respond in the same way as it did in our youth. But we also have to accept that we should put in some effort to get back near to that point if we want to regain the energy we once had. If we don't try, we aid the ageing process, and tempt the fate associated with a high level of metabolically-inactive fat around the stomach—the older man's Achilles heel.

Evolution and the taste for fat

There is another thing that evolution has done—or not done—for us which doesn't help an expanding middle: we have a taste for fat. Many people have a 'fat tooth' (rather than a 'sweet tooth') which gives them a craving for high-calorie foods. And while this is fine when there's not a lot of food around, it can be counter-productive when there is.

Professor Kerin O'Dea from Deakin University in Melbourne calls this 'the land of milk and honey' effect. She claims that human beings evolved at a time when a craving for fat increased the potential to store more energy in case a shortage was coming up. This excess was then 'run off' in running after or working for that fat. A gram of fat yields 9 Calories (37kJ) of energy whereas a gram of carbohydrate provides only 4

Calories (16kJ). So a diet higher in fats results in more energy reserve for the lean times.

It's really only over the last 50–60 years that we have had free access to a wide variety of processed foods. Because a craving for fat is probably inherent, manufacturers have had a heyday selling us food products that are high in fat and refined sugars (another concentrated source of energy). We don't have to chase our food to catch it any more, so we don't burn up energy on that side of the equation. The result could be nature's answer to the 'land of milk and honey', population control through the early demise of those members of the species who become overfat. Charles Darwin claimed that life was based on the survival of the fittest, not the fattest.

It's these two effects of civilisation—increased fat in the diet and the decreased need to have to chase it—that have probably been responsible for most of the self-induced health problems that are common today. This shows up not only in levels of disease, but also in less tangible ways such as lack of well-being, decreased levels of energy and reduced feelings of control over one's life.

The two effects of civilisation—increased fat in the diet and the decreased need to have to chase it—have probably been responsible for most of the self-induced health problems of today.

Professor O'Dea has spent many years studying nutrition in tribal societies such as the Australian Aborigines. She supports claims that those societies who have survived for millennia on low-fat, high-fibre diets tend to have a 'thrifty gene'. This helps them store fat to get through the bad times more easily than European and other Western cultures. However, when such cultures are faced with the 'land of milk and honey' syndrome in a society with readily available processed foods and alcohol, the 'thrifty gene' system breaks down. There is an increase in belly fat and a change in blood sugars and the insulin which helps these sugars to be used as energy with the result that diabetes, heart disease and gallstones—all diseases of modern abdominal obesity—occur at a much faster rate than in non-native peoples.

Medical researchers now think that, in men, the build-up of fat around the middle is the first stage of a range of problems known as 'syndrome X' which is highly predictive of heart disease, diabetes and a range of other metabolic disorders. In syndrome X blood sugar levels and blood fats (cholesterol and triglycerides) are high and blood pressure is raised—all of these are related to a 'pot belly'. In fact, a pot belly measured by a high 'waist-to-hip' ratio is usually a good predictor of syndrome X and therefore of impending health problems.

GB high energy tip

Count fat not calories. It's fat calories that are most damaging to fatness as well as fitness. So calorie counting is out, and fat counting is in.

The symptoms and possible outcomes of syndrome X

Symptoms	Possible health outcomes
Hypertension (high blood pressure)	Heart disease/stroke
Hyperlipidemia (high blood fats)	Diabetes
Hyperglycemia (high blood sugars)	Some cancers (e.g. bowel)
Abdominal obesity	Gallstones

Body shapes

We all have different body shapes. Life wouldn't be very interesting if we were all the same. Our body shapes are largely dictated by heredity. Some people are short and stocky, others long and lean. Not everyone can expect to be trim, taut and terrific and it's not the function of this program to suggest that this can be the case. Whatever the basic body shape, it's the ability to store fat (albeit at different rates) and the resulting excess fat—not the underlying body shape—which can be unhealthy. In a man, excess fat on the stomach is particularly unhealthy and has now been shown to be a good predictor of many different types of disease as well as an indication of low levels of fitness and general poor health. Modern industrialised society is ideal for the development of this type of fatness and lack of fitness. So modern man is in need of methods to cope with this. The GutBuster 'Waist Loss' Program was designed to handle the fatness in a way that is least likely to cause disruption to the enjoyment of modern living. The GutBuster High Energy Program is designed to continue that process by concentrating on other aspects of health and well-being in men—an area that has been long neglected.

3 Not whether, but *how* men and women are different

There was a time when men were men, women were women, and anyone else had trouble buying clothes off the rack! Now, it's often difficult to argue that there are any such things as 'sex differences'. If it wasn't for the obvious appendage dissimilarities, there would be no need for separate bathrooms.

Yet there's mounting evidence that men and women *are* different, if in no other way than the way in which they store, gain and lose body fat. As any discerning female who has ever undergone a fat loss program with a male consort knows, women do it tougher. There's no question about it. The only question until now, has been 'why'? And what does this mean in terms of waist loss programs for men, such as the GutBuster Program?

There are two main reasons why it's easier for men to lose body fat. The first is psychological, the second physiological (we could possibly also add a third, 'sociological', and so cover the whole gamut). Psychologically, as well as physiologically, men and women are almost like different sub-species of the same animal. Men, so it is said, do things *and then think about them*; women think about things *and then do them*. In general, it could be argued that men seek success early in life and then look for meaning while women seek meaning and then look for success.

It is this knowledge in women who have tried dieting, plus the pressure put on females to attain the mythical 'perfect figure', that makes fat loss in women a psychological problem. Cognitive (thought) patterns have been so adversely structured over the years that belief systems in women have developed in a way that acts against long-term fat loss. Many women believe, for example, that they are not worthy because they are

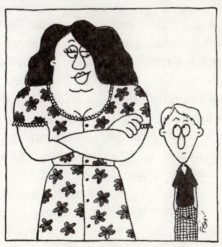

HoMoSexuS 2050.

not able to keep fat off over a long period of time and
that this means that they are also unworthy in other
aspects of life. In psychologist Dr Martin Seligman's
terms, they regard their failures in weight control as
permanent, *pervasive* and *personal*. Any effort to
achieve fat loss goals in women must first deal with
these thought processes, before considering techniques
of simple behaviour change—such as food restriction
and exercise—that might lead to fat loss.

---

*Like bulls in a paddock, men fatten
up in the good times and thin out
in the bad times. This varies
according to the amount and type of
fatty food available and is inversely
proportional to the amount of
exercise required to get that food.*

Men, on the other hand, are quite simple beings
(some might say too simple). Their corpulence in modern
society is largely a result of things simply being too easy.
Fatness is a behavioural problem in most men, not
necessarily a cognitive one. Like bulls in a paddock, they
fatten up in the good times and thin out in the bad times.
This varies according to the amount and type of fatty
food available and is inversely proportional to the
amount of exercise required to get that food.

Changing behaviour, or 'behaviour modification' as
psychologists call it, is much more simple than changing
thought patterns. Fat loss in men, therefore, is a
relatively easy process once they've made up their
minds.

GB high energy tip

Monitor changes in behaviour and feelings of wellness, not just changes in waist size. Most people underestimate the food they eat and overestimate the exercise they do. Recording this shows you the actual case.

Different types of fat

The difference in psychological patterning between men and women is also helped by differences in physiology. Men, as we've seen repeatedly, store fat around the stomach. The fat cells in this part of the body are different in size and much more 'lypolytic'—meaning that they give up their fat more readily for energy— than fat cells in lower parts of the body. The pot belly can therefore be thought of as a giant water bag that men carry around with them for periods of drought. It is pretty easy to empty out a water bag. You just tip it up, or dry it out with heat.

In women, the fat cells situated around the hips, buttocks and thighs are smaller than those around the stomach and much more resistant to fat loss because they are there for reproductive purposes. We know that this type of fat becomes even more resistant under conditions of starvation or excessive exercise. These fat cells are more like the reserve fuel tank in an old VW. The fuel from these is only used as a last resource. You can't just tip them up or dry them out at will.

There's a range of evidence which now shows quite clearly that physiological differences between males and females work against females burning up fat as easily as males. For example, the enzyme lipoprotein lipase

Some facts of life—from a male perspective

- The average Australian man lives six years less than the average woman.
- Longevity for higher-income males is still lower than that for lower-income females.
- The death rate for men is higher than women at all ages after 15.
- In the 1920s excess male over female mortality was 20 per cent. In 1990 it was 70 per cent.
- Men suffer twice the rate of heart disease, one-and-a-half times the rate of respiratory disorders and up to twice the rate of cancer as women.
- Men at all ages are twice as likely to die from injury or violence as women.
- Around 48 per cent of men are regarded as over-weight or obese compared to 33 per cent of women.
- Men use Medicare 30 per cent less than women.
- Men are more likely than women to drink, smoke and engage in other unhealthy activities.
- The federal government has provided $205 million for breast cancer research over 5 years. Research for testicular and prostate cancer (which kill as many men as breast cancers kill women) has received no extra funding.

(LPL), which helps store fat in fat cells, is much more active in female lower body fat cells than in the upper body cells of men. On the other hand, the enzyme 'hormone stimulating lipase' (HSL), which helps break down fat, is less active in lower body fat cells of women.

The female hormone 'oestrogen' is also indirectly involved in lower body fat storage, whereas the male sex hormones or 'androgens' are more involved in upper body, and particularly waist, fat storage. Females also have a lower lean body mass (muscle) content than men and because muscle is active, whereas fat is passive, this means that men burn more energy at rest than women. The male metabolic rate is, therefore, naturally higher than that for a woman and the higher muscle content means a greater energy use for a given amount of exercise. It may seem unfair to a woman, but walking a kilometre will burn more calories for most men than it will for most women.

Differences in the female shape—larger hips, more fat and a lower centre of gravity—also mean that some exercises, such as swimming, are much less fat burning for women than for men. Their higher body fat content and lower centre of gravity means they are *more* efficient in the water (strangely, a disadvantage—see Chapter 9) and, therefore, burn less energy. Men, being more muscle dense, tend to sink more—like a stone— and therefore have to use more energy to stay afloat.

Finally, thermogenesis, or heat loss, which is also a source of energy burning, is greater in men because of the higher muscle mass. Thermogenesis increases after a meal and is likely to have a greater effect in men than in women. All these factors are summarised in Table 3.1.

Fat sociology

That's not the end of the story. As well as the psychological and the physiological differences, we have to add on the effects of social pressures and their outcomes. The pressure on women to diet over the years, particularly in adolescence, has led to problems with weight cycling. Rapid loss then rapid gain has long-term

Table 3.1 Male–female differences in fat storage and fat loss

Males	Females
Fat stored mainly around the stomach	Fat stored mainly on hips and buttocks
Fat cells larger	Fat cells smaller
Fat 'burned' up more readily	Fat not 'burned' up so readily
More energy burned for a given amount of exercise	Less energy burned for a given amount of exercise
Fat less resistant to exercises such as swimming	Fat more resistant to exercises such as swimming (because of support in water given by a higher percentage body fat)
Fat used up more easily to compensate for fasting	Fat more resistant to fasting
Less risk of weight cycling	More risk of weight cycling
Fat levels unaffected by reproduction	Fat levels may be increased following several pregnancies
High thermogenic (heat loss) effect following food intake	Lower thermogenic effect following food intake
More energy used for metabolism (and therefore natural energy burning)	Less energy used for metabolism (and therefore natural fat storage)

consequences on metabolism. Men have fewer problems with cycling. They seem to steadily put fat on from their early twenties until such time as they want to take it off. They usually take fat off once they decide to get serious. The pressures on women are to be thin. As Marlene Dietrich once said 'A woman can never be too rich or too thin'. Everything is directed towards that end. Women don't aim to be fit or healthy or more energetic—they aim to be thin. At the extreme, we see the eating disorders bulimia and anorexia nervosa, which now afflict up to 5–10 per cent of the female population. The ideal body image for most men, on the other hand, is not to be thin, but to have bulk. You could hardly compare Arnold Schwarzenegger with Twiggy! Some female psychologists working in the area of weight control are now concerned that new pressures on men to lose weight will mean that more men will also develop anorexia. But the evidence points the other way. Most men seek bulk, because it is this which offers power, masculinity and a message of protection in the mating game.

Everything, it seems, works against the female in fat loss. But before women feel too bad about that, they should remember the swings and roundabouts. Lower-body fat stores in women have few known adverse health consequences, apart from, perhaps, a slight increase in the risk of varicose veins and arthritis. Upper body, or abdominal, fat in men however, is clearly associated with an increased risk of heart disease, diabetes, some cancers and a whole range of other health problems.

This, then, links back to our original suggestion that fat loss is more of a psychological issue for females and a behavioural issue for males. The fact is, men and women *are* different. In matters of body fat they're like

---

GB high energy tip

Avoid dieting or fasting. These forms of masochism were devised (unsuccessfully) for female weight control. They have no place in men's (or women's) health.

two different species—mice and rats if you like (and we'll leave it to the reader to determine which is which). No matter how much some feminist groups would like to dispute this, the conclusion remains, in health as well as in fat loss—sex differences do exist. Vive la différence!

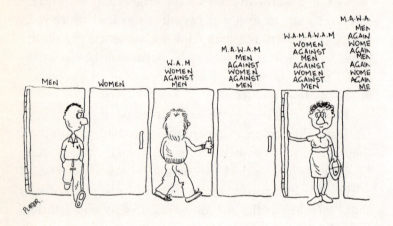

4 Repeating the GutBuster principles

In the *GutBuster Waist Loss Guide*, we outlined four basic principles for effective waist loss. Before proceeding to discuss high level energy, these need to be restated. In summary, they are as follows:

1 Changing habits.
2 Moving more.
3 Eating differently (particularly less fat and more fibre).
4 Trading off (food and drink for exercise).

We'll summarise each of these to refresh your memory.

Changing habits

Habits are ways of responding that become automatic—we have stopped thinking about what we are doing and why. Habits form from a connection between a stimulus and a response. That stimulus is not always hunger but

29

can be the cues that we've learned to associate with eating. For example, an advertisement during a television program can come to be associated with getting up and finding something to eat or drink. It's the advertisement, not the hunger, that leads to excessive eating. To break this 'habit' cycle, the stimulus–response connection needs to be broken. Some tips for doing this are outlined below and a more detailed list is given in Chapter 12.

'Stalking' habits and changing stimulus–response (S–R) connections are the main implications of focusing on the role of habits in waist control. These are considered in more depth in 'Trading off' below.

Tips for changing eating habits

- Identify triggers for eating.
- Measure waist size weekly and record it.
- Focus on your behaviour rather than your weight.
- Don't keep high-fat snack foods (chocolates, chips, biscuits etc.) in the house.
- *Never* shop while hungry.
- Confine eating to one place in the house (such as the dining room table).
- Leave the table immediately after eating.
- Don't associate anything else, such as reading or TV, with eating.
- Wait for five minutes in the middle of a meal before eating more.
- Don't get into a 'shout'.
- Substitute an alternative for eating, like going for a walk or washing the car.
- Combine water/mineral water chasers with alcohol.
- Reward yourself for *doing* things, not just *achieving* things.

Moving more

Most fat control programs emphasise diet. But more and more people are beginning to recognise the import- ance of movement or exercise. The first point to make about exercise for fatness is that it's not necessarily the same as exercising for fitness. In fact, exercise is the wrong term. All you need is more movement. Move- ment of any kind uses up energy. And energy, as we know, if not taken in in the form of food, is taken out of the body in the form of fat.

A planned exercise or fitness program will obviously burn fat, but you don't have to go to a gym or take up aerobics, or even pound the pavement in a pair of joggers. Moving more might simply mean walking a bit more instead of going everywhere in the car, becoming a little more active with the kids or mowing the lawn instead of paying someone else to do it.

So let's forget 'bust-a-gut exercise' and think about moving more, in big ways and little ways, all the time throughout the day (see next page).

More tips on movement and why long, gentle, continuous movement is the optimum for fat loss are considered in Part III: Making the most of movement.

Eating differently

Losing fat doesn't necessarily mean eating less—it means eating differently. In particular, it means decreas- ing fat in the diet and increasing fibre.

Decreasing fat in the diet

One gram of fat provides your body with 9 Calories

Tips for moving more

- Try to walk every day (at least six days a week) for at least 3–4 kms.
- Park away from a restaurant or shop or work and walk to and from it.
- Go for a walk or drink water instead of automatically snacking.
- Have an alternative exercise planned for cold/wet days.
- Organise a friend or partner to exercise with you so that you can't renege.
- If injury stops you from walking, try a bike, swimming, a mini-tramp—anything.
- Don't do any organised exercise you don't like for longer than two weeks.
- Exercise *before* a main meal. With the exception of swimming, exercise reduces the appetite.
- Vary your exercise (either different exercises each day or a different route each day).
- Plan ahead, and make sure that you don't miss out on moving for at least two consecutive days.
- Don't use a lift or escalator when you can use the stairs.
- Don't ride when you can walk.

(37kJ), whereas a gram of either carbohydrate or protein has only 4 Calories (17kJ). So fat is more fattening. It also seems to be more addictive, so the more fat we eat, the more we crave it. You can reduce fat, and hence the craving for fat and food in the following ways:

1 Trim all fat off meat.
2 Remove skin from chicken.
3 Choose fish or other seafood.
4 Buy lean meat and poultry, e.g. skinless chicken legs, breasts or thighs.

5 Cook with less fat by:
- grilling;
- microwaving;
- dry frying;
- barbecuing;
- steaming.
6 Choose low fat (cottage, or ricotta) or reduced-fat cheeses.
7 Use spreads thinly—or skip them altogether.
8 Buy low-fat dairy products—skim or lite milk and low-fat yoghurt.
9 Keep cakes, biscuits, pies, take-aways, pastry and toasted muesli to a minimum.

Increasing fibre

Dietary fibre is found in plant foods. Fibre tends to create a 'full' feeling so that you feel satisfied. High-fibre foods are rarely fattening, mainly because they are bulky so it is difficult to eat too much of them. Some hints for adding fibre to your diet are:

1 Use wholemeal bread.
2 Choose wholegrain cereals such as wholemeal pasta, brown rice, wholegrain crispbread, rolled oats, and wheat, barley or oat breakfast cereals.
3 Eat the skins of fruits and vegetables where appropriate.
4 Eat more vegetables and fruit.
5 Eat more dried peas, beans and lentils (e.g. soy beans, kidney beans, baked beans, Lima beans etc.).
6 Eat fibre with protein (a chicken and salad sandwich—not just chicken).

Decreasing fat and increasing fibre are the two main changes that can help in the early stages of a fat loss program. Sugars, although usually given great importance in many programs, really only need to be considered once fats are under control. In this book we consider sugar in Chapter 8.

Trading off

For many men, the idea of not being able to enjoy a drink often stops them from trying to reduce their gut. But there's a good reason for trying to cut down. Every gram of alcohol is equivalent to 7 Calories (29kJ) (water has no calories). Alcohol may also slow down the rate at which fat is burned in the body. And because it doesn't take much energy to convert fat in the blood to storage fat, the effects of alcohol can mean that even more fat gets deposited on the belly. So, instead of fat in the diet being used as energy, it fills the fat cell reservoirs around the waist.

Fortunately, you don't have to give up all of the good things in life. What's the point in making your life miserable? You can enjoy a drink *and* lose waist but to be able to do so, you'll need to make some trade offs in the type of food you eat and the amount of movement you do. As a rough guide, one middie of beer needs you to walk or jog about 1.5 kilometres

---

GB high energy tip

Walk at least 1 km for each alcoholic drink. Speed is not important. Walk 3–4 kms per day—more if desired.

(about a mile), although the effect of exercise on metabolic rate may reduce this distance slightly. We can say that you need to walk one extra kilometre for each alcoholic drink. It's a small price to pay. Alternatively, a middie of beer is equivalent to a couple of biscuits or a small piece of cake. To balance out up to 4 beers a day, you can decrease the amount of biscuits, cake or other fatty foods you eat, or increase your walking.

Trading off is a simple way of doing things which have a big effect on waist reduction while not having to drastically alter your lifestyle. We've discussed some techniques before. We'll look at some others throughout this book.

A guide to the high energy way

The GutBuster High Energy Program builds on the initial *GutBuster Waist Loss Guide*, but it is not intended to replace it. Indeed, the information contained in the earlier guide should be seen as a base for this new material. Although significant gains could be made using just the principles outlined here, these gains will be much more effective over the long term if this program is added to the first. Information changes so rapidly and the decade of the 1990s is likely to be the decade of men's health, so we don't even see this book as being the end of the story. We do, however, contend that we have provided some of the newest scientific information in the area of fat control. For this reason, this book should be read not as a step-by-step guide, but as an information primer for a total lifestyle 'grease and oil change'. We can also guarantee that you'll come out of it feeling better for being intellectually lubricated.

II

Feeding the fading fatness

5 Why dieting is a waste of good food

Think of *weight* control and most people, especially women, automatically think *diet*. Weight control and diets are almost synonymous. But they are synonymously wrong!

As we've seen, it's not *weight* control so much as *fat* control that is important. Diets that restrict food intake usually cause you to lose *weight* but the lowered figure on the scales that most people use as a mark of success does not discriminate between the types of body tissue that have been lost. We also know that severe calorie restriction predisposes people to binge eating and also sets the scene for regaining weight more easily at a later stage. Very low calorie diets are really a form of semi-starvation. With each dieting episode, the rate of fat loss is slower, and once you return to normal eating, the regain is faster. Let's look at the reasons why.

With strict diets that cut down drastically on calories, the body burns not only fat but muscle. Loss of muscle and loss of muscle glycogen (the energy stores within the muscle) also cause a massive loss of water from the body. The water will return once you go back to eating normally, but the muscle tissue will not magically reappear. Muscle is biologically active tissue that burns up calories even when resting, so its loss means that the body can no longer burn up as many calories as before.

If you fast (or starve), about 85 per cent of the *weight* lost is water and much of the remainder is lean muscle tissue. For every gram of muscle energy (glycogen) or muscle protein lost, the body releases about three grams of water. That's largely responsible for the so-called *weight* loss on most dieting programs. It is not *fat* loss. Very low calorie diets are not much better than starvation and they cause a greater loss of water and muscle than body fat.

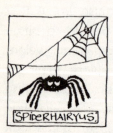
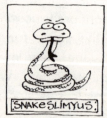
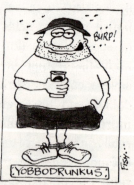

THE AUSTRALIAN WOMAN'S MOST HATED SPECIES COLLECTION

Low calorie diets and muscle loss

If someone follows a very low calorie diet for life, they'll lose *weight* but the rate of weight loss will taper off as the body reduces its muscle and so needs fewer calories. In theory, if you kept to a very low calorie diet, you'd continue to lose *weight,* even though at a reduced rate. In practice, almost no one could follow a very low calorie diet for life and, once a dieter returns to eating normally, weight gain follows. With less muscle tissue, the amount of food which once kept that person's weight steady will now cause an increase, simply because the loss of muscle from the body has reduced the number of calories the body can burn.

We can demonstrate this with some simple arithmetic. Let's say that metabolic rate accounts for 1700 Calories (7140 kJ) a day (a typical level in an average-sized man) and food intake is around 2200 Calories (9240 kJ) a day. To maintain a balance with no excess calories left for storage, 500 Calories (2100 kJ) need to be burned in normal day-to-day activity. If we introduce a 1200 Calorie (5040 kJ) a day diet, our man is taking in 500 fewer calories than his metabolism requires, so he'll lose weight. If he doesn't exercise, his weight loss will be from lean tissue (muscle) as well as some fat. The muscle loss however will decrease his metabolic rate. If we assume that his resting metabolic rate decreases by about 15 per cent (a common decrease after a loss of even 2 kg of muscle), he'll now need only 1450 Calories (6090 kJ) a day for metabolism. When he goes back to his normal 2200 Calories a day, he must now expend 750 Calories (3150 kJ) a day in activity to avoid storing excess calories as fat. Since his normal day-to-day activity uses only 500 Calories, he's now left with 250 spare Calories (1050 kJ). These will be stored as fat and could result in a gain of 1 kg of fat every 30 days, or 12 kg of extra fat each year. (These figures are only theoretical and will vary for different individuals.) Had our hapless porcine followed an even stricter diet—women's magazine style or popular diet book type—he would reduce his muscle by an even greater amount and would regain weight even faster!

For every gram of muscle energy (glycogen) or muscle protein lost, the body releases about three grams of water. That's largely responsible for the so-called weight loss on most dieting programs. It's not fat loss.

The loss of muscle and the consequent reduction in metabolic rate is a major argument *against* dieting, and it's especially relevant for fasting or strict diets that promise fast weight loss. Studies show that slower weight loss is less likely to lead to loss of muscle and reduction in metabolic rate.

But reducing metabolic rate is not the only bad feature of diets. *Going on* a diet implies that you will one day *come off* it. Unless you've learned new eating habits that you can live with, fat loss won't be permanent. Any changes you make must be maintained for a lifetime. They must therefore be changes that are enjoyable and fit in with your lifestyle. If you party all the time, you need to learn habits that fit in with parties. If you travel, your new habits must be compatible with what you can achieve. Dieting could be regarded as a severe form of masochism. But, in spite of this, and the known high failure rate with diets, diet 'experts' continue to preach the gospel of dieting, even though they know that few people will ever stick to diets, let alone enjoy them. Dieting is therefore usually a waste of good food.

We propose instead that you make small changes in the amount of fat you eat because we believe that this can be done without losing the enjoyment of eating well. Most people aren't even aware of much of the fat they eat and choosing different foods with less fat will not be a great hardship. Exercise can also be enjoyable and some people even find it a positive addiction (as Garry Egger has described in his book *The Sport Drug*, Allen & Unwin, Sydney, 1982). When something gives such positive feedback, it is much more likely to be continued over the long term, and therefore has a greater chance of success.

What about food intake?

Reducing energy intake, along with moving more, is also important to reduce body fat. If you do enough exercise you may be able to give up worrying about energy intake from food and drinks, especially once you've reduced your body fat to reasonable levels. Athletes after all, often eat two to four times as much as ordinary people and still stay lean.

So how can you reduce energy intake without

dieting? The answer is simple. Change the *type* of foods you eat. Fats have the highest calorie level (9 Cal/g, 37 kJ/g) whereas proteins and carbohydrates are much lower (4 Cal/g, 17 kJ/g). Fibre has even fewer calories because it's digested by bacteria in the large intestine and there's some loss of calories to the bacteria themselves. By reducing fat and increasing fibre, it's possible to end up eating *more* food while taking in *less* energy. It's also a pattern you can follow for a lifetime because it doesn't mean that you're going to go hungry. If you allow yourself to become very hungry, you're likely to eat the first thing that comes along, irrespective of whether it's something you really want or not. As often as not, spur-of-the moment food choices tend to be high-fat foods. The GutBuster Program suggests that you never go for more than four hours without something to eat and if you get hungry before that, you can always have some high-fibre, low-fat food.

To add to the beneficial effects of low-fat, high-fibre foods (for a detailed list of these, see *GutBuster Waist Loss Guide*), you can also reduce the amount of sugar you eat. Carbohydrates don't increase fat levels, but eating too many will provide your body with enough energy so that it won't get round to burning its fat

---

GB high energy tip

Never go for more than four hours without something to eat. Control over the *type* of food you eat is much more difficult when you're hungry. So eat some high-fibre, low-fat food *before* you get hungry.

supply so well. As we've mentioned already, you're unlikely to eat too many of the high-fibre, complex carbohydrate foods because they're so filling. Sugar is another kettle of fish because you *can* overdo it more easily. High-fibre foods also supply other important nutrients whereas sugar has none, so your body won't suffer at all if you eat less of it.

Fat loss and high-energy wellness has to be a way of life and an enjoyable way of life for it to last. Dieting is not only not enjoyable, it's often downright stupid! We hope that foolish diets will eventually disappear as more people recognise that they don't work. If they did work, there wouldn't need to be a new one almost every week!

We're also concerned about the proliferation of weight control powdered products, often sold through networks of friends and acquaintances. Most of these fit into the worst category of all diets—they're very low in calories, very low in fibre and contribute very little bulk. Some contain small amounts of fibre that are supposed to swell inside the stomach to give a 'full' feeling. Others contain herbs which are endowed with almost magic properties. In fact, most of the herbs turn out to be laxatives which increase the loss of water—not fat—from the body. They're worse than useless, as any weight loss is unlikely to be permanent; they're not products that you can use for a lifetime; and they have the potential to increase the risk of bowel cancer. Persuasive salespeople may extol their virtues, but our advice is to stop believing in fairy stories!

A lifetime of changes, or changes for a lifetime

Weight control programs, especially those designed to appeal to women, lead to a lifetime of changes—on again, off again; thin one month, fat the next, then thin again. These continual changes to the body's metabolism confuse it so that, over the long term, it gradually slows down. Metabolic rate decreases over the dieting period, then rises in between diets. The rate of weight loss declines with repeated dieting, as we've seen, mainly because the proportion of total body mass, that is fat, increases while muscle decreases.

In women, the off–on–off–on weight pattern is sometimes called the *rhythm method of girth control* (see graph). It's common in young women who alternate crash dieting or semi-starvation with binge eating

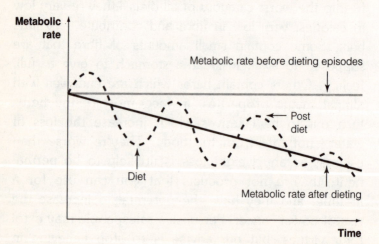

Metabolic rate

Metabolic rate before dieting episodes

Post diet

Diet

Metabolic rate after dieting

Time

The rhythm method of girth control

at a stage in their life cycle when their metabolism is establishing its permanent adult level.

We must repeat that permanent fat loss means changes for a lifetime. The GutBuster Program therefore states that anything that is done in the name of waist reduction must be enjoyable, whether it be changing food habits or exercising. If it's not enjoyable, you can't do it for a lifetime. And if it can't be maintained for a lifetime, it won't work.

It's important to read this book in that context. If a suggested exercise is something that you either hate doing or can't do, find an alternative. If cutting back on the booze interferes with your lifestyle, trade it off against some of the other suggested changes. If some food is particularly important to you, you can trade it off for something else. Not only do you not have to *bust a gut to lose a gut*, you have to have a good *gut feeling* for what you're doing.

GB high energy tip

Don't make changes that you can't maintain for a lifetime. Changes that are likely to be temporary, like cutting back on the grog, or 'going on a diet', mean that any fat loss or health effects are also likely to be temporary.

---

6 Finding out about fats

Fats are usually thought of as being the bad guys of nutrition. But this is not true for all fats. Some are essential in the diet and make up part of the structure of all body cells. Particular fatty acids are important in nerve and brain cells and in specialised tissues such as the retina of the eye. Some fatty acids from foods are used as building blocks for the body to make hormone-like substances called prostaglandins. These influence (among other things) blood pressure, the way blood clots, how we react to injury and inflammation in tissues, and the body's response to infection. Fats are also important sources of energy in the body, especially for growing babies and children.

Fats are made up of fatty acids and a substance called glycerol. It's the fatty acids that are of greatest interest because it's differences in these that make fats either desirable or dispensable in the diet. The chem-

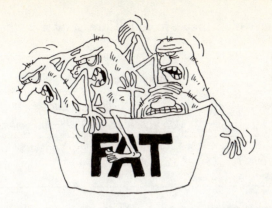

istry of fats is complicated but we'll try to explain some of the more basic aspects as simply as possible. If you don't want to know about this, it won't hurt to skip to the end of this chapter. For fat loss, all you really need to know is that we currently think that all fats have equal numbers of calories and all types should be reduced. Oils are just different types of fats in liquid form and the same rules apply to these in relation to fat loss. In terms of health, it is the *type* of fat which is most important and information about this forms the basis of the next part of this chapter.

Fats in foods can be divided into two major categories: saturated and unsaturated. Within the unsaturated category, there are also two major classes: mono-unsaturated and polyunsaturated. The types of fats and the

---

GB high energy tip

Keep all fats and oils in the diet to less than 40 g a day. All fats and oils, regardless of type, are equally fattening. Add up your fat intake with a fat counter like Rosemary Stanton's 'Fat and Fibre Counter'.

forms in which they are found are shown in the table below:

Fatty acids

Saturated	Unsaturated	
	Mono-unsaturated	Polyunsaturated
Meats	Olive oils	Vegetable oils
Coconut oil	Canola oil	
Dairy fats		

What do fatty acids look like?

A fatty acid molecule comprises a chain of carbon atoms with hydrogen atoms attached as shown in Figure 6.1 below. The end of the molecule with three hydrogens attached to the carbon atom is known as the methyl end. The other end is known as the carboxyl end. The chain usually has an even number of carbon atoms which stretches from four to 24 carbon atoms. In general, if there are less than 10 carbons in the chain, the fatty acid is called a *short chain* fatty acid. These are commonly found in dairy fats. If there are 12, 14, 16 or 18 carbon atoms, the fatty acid is called a *medium chain* fat. These are commonly found in chocolate, meat and processed fats. Fatty acids with more than 20 carbons are called *long chain* fatty acids and are found in breast milk, seafoods and some seeds and vegetables. Medium chain fatty acids are changed within the body to longer chain fatty acids.

Saturated fats

If every carbon atom has its full complement of hydro-

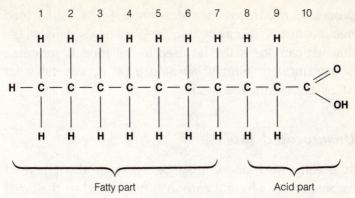

Figure 6.1 **Structure of a saturated fatty acid**

gen atoms attached, the fat is *saturated*, meaning that it has as many hydrogen atoms as it can possibly hold. The most commonly occurring saturated fatty acids have 10, 12, 14, 16 or 18 carbon atoms in their chains and are found in meats, dairy products, chocolate, processed fats, coconut and palm kernel oils. Saturated fats are *not* found only in animal products, as is sometimes believed. Much of the saturated fat in our diet now comes from processed foods and originates from vegetable sources such as palm kernel oil. When you see the words 'vegetable oil' on the label of a food product, it may well be a saturated vegetable oil with little health benefit. The fatty acid shown in Figure 6.1 is a saturated fat.

Saturated fats are usually solid at room temperature (such as dripping, butter or chocolate). They keep fairly well and this makes them attractive to food manufacturers. They also make crisp biscuits and pastry and crunchy coatings on fried food. Because they're cheap, have a relatively long shelf-life and are useful in processed foods, saturated fats are widely used by food manufacturers. Improved food labelling is needed so that we can see if the fat used in the food is saturated or unsaturated. Simply labelling a fat as vegetable fat or oil is of little real value.

Unsaturated fats

In a fatty acid, there may be spots in the chain of carbon atoms where a carbon is not bound to the usual number of hydrogen atoms. In such cases, the spare carbon, like every lonely soul, is looking for a partner, and forms a double bond with its next-door carbon neighbour. If there is only one double bond in the molecule, it looks like the molecule shown in Figure 6.2 and is called a *mono-unsaturated* fatty acid (MUFA). The most common mono-unsaturated fat has 18 carbon atoms, with the double bond occurring on the ninth carbon atom from the methyl end of the

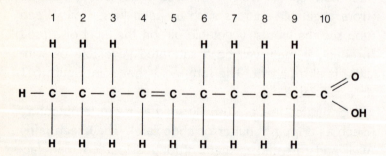

Figure 6.2   *Structure of a mono-unsaturated fatty acid*

chain. It's known as oleic acid and it is one of the most abundant fatty acids, being the principal fatty acid in olive and canola oils.

If there's more than one double bond in the fatty acid, the structure may look like that shown in Figure 6.3. These are called *polyunsaturated* fatty acids (PUFA). The most common source of polyunsaturated fatty acids are oils such as sunflower, safflower, corn, sesame, soy bean and grapeseed. Some special types of very long chain polyunsaturated fats are found in fish and in breast milk.

Omega 3 and omega 6

Polyunsaturated fats are also categorised according to where the double bonds occur along the carbon chain. If the first double bond occurs on the third carbon from the methyl end of the carbon chain, the fatty acid is called an omega 3 fatty acid (also written as n–3). These polyunsaturated fatty acids occur in fish and all seafoods

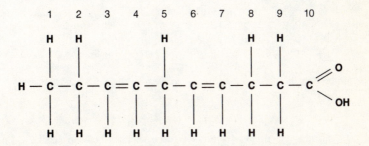

Figure 6.3   Structure of a polyunsaturated fat

and also in some seeds and in breast milk. They have become popular lately as 'healthy oils' which help prevent heart disease. If the first double bond occurs on the sixth carbon from the methyl end of the chain, it is known as an omega 6 fatty acid (also written as n–6). The polyunsaturated fats in the vegetable oils mentioned earlier, and also in the margarines made from these oils, are the omega 6 type. Evening primrose oil is also an omega 6 fatty acid.

There are specific rules for describing fatty acids according to their structure and the position of their double bonds. In Figure 6.3, the double bonds occur on the third and sixth carbon atoms from the methyl end of the carbon chain. This was a hypothetical fatty acid, but if it existed it could be written in shorthand as C10:2n–3 because it has 10 carbons (C10), two double bonds (:2) and the first double bond occurs on the third carbon from the end (n–3).

Omega 3s and 6s are often in the news because nutritionists now believe they need to be present in the diet in the right balance. If not (and this is often the

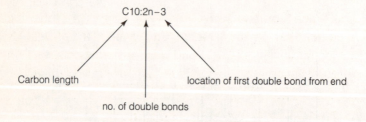

Shorthand for a 'family' of fats with a double bond of 3 carbon atoms from the methyl end of the chain (also called an omega 3 fatty acid).

Figure 6.4   *Conventional naming of fatty acids*

case in many modern diets), they compete with each other to use up an enzyme which both need for their metabolism within the body. The two major players in this competition are an omega 6 fatty acid called linoleic acid (C18:2n–6) and an omega 3 fatty acid called linolenic acid (C18:3n–3). Both are essential for humans but if we have too much linoleic, the body is unable to deal with linolenic acid properly. Polyunsaturated oils and margarines are high in linoleic acid and can create problems if they are eaten in large quantities. It is commonly thought that it is a good thing to eat polyunsaturated fats, but it's a case of too much of a good thing is a nuisance.

Oleic acid (C18:n–9), the mono-unsaturated fatty acid found in olive and canola oils, has its only double bond on the ninth carbon from the methyl end of the chain. It does not compete with the other two essential fatty acids and is generally regarded as an all-round good guy.

Cis and trans fatty acids

Just when you thought you had it all worked out, we have another factor to take into account. Fatty acids that contain a double bond can align themselves in different geometric formations. If the hydrogen atoms

---

GB high energy tip

Eat seafood (but not fried) at least 1–2 times per week. All seafood (yes, even prawns) are relatively low in fat and high in healthy (omega 3) oils.

attached to the carbons that have formed a double bond with each other are on the same side of the molecule, as shown below, the molecule is known as a *cis* fatty acid. If the hydrogen atoms are on opposite sides, then the fatty acid is called *trans*.

The cis or trans configuration determines the fate of the molecule within the body. The picture is also complicated by the number of carbon atoms involved in the fatty acid. Trans fatty acids that occur in dairy products, for example, have fewer carbon atoms than the trans fatty acids formed when polyunsaturated fats are processed. It's only the trans fatty acids formed during heating and processing that give cause for concern. These fats are now thought to be unhealthy and they have tarnished the previous halo that was placed over polyunsaturated fats. Most polyunsaturated margarines, for example, contain about 12 per cent trans fatty acids.

Recent research shows that trans fatty acids from processed fats may not 'fit' the areas of the body they

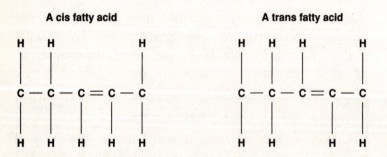

Figure 6.5   Fatty acids

Summary

Fats and oils have a number of variable components that alter their nature and healthful properties. These include:

1 The length of the carbon chain (*long*, *medium* or *short* chain fatty acids).
2 The presence or absence of double bonds (*unsaturated* or *saturated* fatty acids).
3 The number of double bonds (*mono* or *poly*unsaturated fatty acids).
4 The position of the double bond (*omega 3*, *omega 6* or *omega 9* fatty acids).
5 The position of hydrogen atoms on the same or opposite sides of the double bond (*cis* or *trans* fatty acids).

were destined for, just as a key with a broken section won't fit its normal lock. Trans fatty acids form from the less stable polyunsaturated fatty acids when processed or exposed to heat or light. They are potentially at least as unhealthy as saturated fats.

Fats, health and fat loss

As we have seen, not all fats are bad. Some fatty acids are essential in the diet. To complicate matters a little more, foods contain more than just one fatty acid. For example, we describe olive oil as being a *mono-unsaturated* fat but olive oil also contains polyunsaturated and some saturated fatty acids. Its *predominant* fatty acid is the mono-unsaturated oleic acid, so we describe it by that name. Sometimes descriptions can be misleading. For example, we think of polyunsaturated margarine being just that—polyunsaturated. In fact, as we've mentioned, about 20 per cent of the fat in these products is saturated fat. They also have some mono-unsaturated fatty acids which are 'good' and about 12 per cent of the undesirable trans fatty acids. Their total polyunsaturated fat content makes up just over half the fat they contain hence they are named after their dominant fats.

The percentage of different fatty acids is really only important if the total amount of fat in the food is significant. Let's look at margarine where the total fat content is high—80 per cent. This means that every 100 grams of the yellow spread has 80 grams of total fat. If 20 per cent of this is saturated fat, the quantity of saturated fat in 100 grams of margarine is about 16 grams—quite a large amount. Even a tablespoon of margarine has 3.2 grams of saturated fat. Yet many people happily eat margarine, thinking that it's a healthy product. It certainly has less saturated fat than butter which rates a high 49 grams in every 100 grams (or 10 grams in a tablespoon). But the total fat content and the total calories in both products are equal. A food such as an egg by contrast, has about 6 grams of fat, of which 2 grams is saturated. By eating a tablespoon of margarine on your toast you take in more than one-and-a-half times as much saturated fat as you'd get from an egg!

Even though all fats provide equally high numbers of calories, it's the saturated fats which are regarded as the most dangerous for raising the amount of cholesterol in the blood, leading to more blood clots forming with their potential to block arteries and cause a heart attack. Polyunsaturated fats are better for reducing blood chol-

---

GB high energy tip

Spread butter AND margarine thinly, or not at all. Both spreads are high in fat (about 80%) and therefore both are equally fattening. Eight slices of bread spread with margarine provides a whole day's recommended fat intake.

---

esterol but even they don't get a clean record for other aspects of health. These fats oxidise rapidly, unless you have a high intake of antioxidants, and they are potentially linked with a higher incidence of diabetes in humans and mammary tumours in animals. One large study over many years has shown that those eating the most margarine had the most heart disease. Polyunsaturates can also form nasty substances when heated more than once. Mono-unsaturated fats are probably the best type of fat. They reduce blood cholesterol at least as well as the polyunsaturates, they don't oxidise so readily and they have no links with other health problems. In the case of olive oil, a major source of mono-unsaturated fat, we also have a long history of people safely consuming it. Its major virtue may be not only that it contains a good mix of fatty acids, but that it also contains a wide variety of antioxidants. **But remember, it still contains the same *calories*, gram for gram, as other types of fats or oils.**

Becoming a 'fat detective'

For the waist watcher, the important thing to remember is that all fats and oils, whatever their type, have the same energy density, and all are probably equally fattening. (We say *probably* as some research is being done which suggests that all may be fattening but some may be even more fattening than others.) The main problem for the waist watcher is to know where fats occur in foods.

---

*All fats and oils, whatever their
type, have the same energy density,
and all are equally fattening.*

Some fats in foods are obvious, such as the thick fatty edge on the outside of meat and the white streaks marbled through it, or the fat under the skin of chicken, or butter, margarine, oils and other cooking fats. Some fats, however, are *invisible* and unless you know what goes into the foods you're eating, it's difficult to know exactly how much fat you're taking in. For example, there's a lot of fat in biscuits (including savoury ones), pastries, cakes, coatings on foods such as fish fingers, oven-fried chips, toasted muesli, fast foods and cheeses.

One of the single most effective ways to high level health is to become a 'fat detective'—seeking out fats in foods and learning to avoid them. How do you know where to find fats? Without a special directory (such as Rosemary Stanton's 'Fat and Fibre Counter') the next best way is to learn how to read labels. Labels take some interpreting as the information you need is not always clear. Sometimes it's clouded by confusing statements such as 'no cholesterol'. This term has been used on foods that are high in fats, including saturated fats. Most of the excess cholesterol in the blood comes when the diet is high in saturated fat. The actual cholesterol content of the food is much less important and contributes very little to blood cholesterol. 'No cholesterol' labels have been confusing and hide the real problem. There is now a new code of practice which will help make food labels more honest. This code states that a food that claims to be 'low fat' or 'reduced fat', 'low sugar', 'low salt', 'high fibre' or to have some similar benefit must conform to certain rules.

For example, 'reduced-fat' foods must not have more than three-quarters of the fat content of regular foods in the same category. Food manufacturers will also have to compare like food with like. A reduced-fat chicken sausage must therefore be compared with a regular sausage made from chicken, not with a meat pie or sausage roll or a salami sausage made from beef.

A 'low-fat' claim on a label will mean the food must not have more than 3 g of fat in every 100 g of food, or half that level for liquid foods, since they are usually consumed in larger amounts.

'Fat free' will mean that only negligible amounts of fat are present while any food whose label states 'x% fat-free' must fit the category of a low-fat food *and* the actual fat content must also be listed. This will put an end to labels making absurd claims such as '85% fat-free'—only those foods that meet the claim for low-fat foods (that is with less than 3 g of fat in 100 g) will be able to claim they are 97, 98, or 99% fat-free.

It would still make it a lot easier if manufacturers told us the fat content of the food rather than this somewhat absurd idea that part of the food is fat-free. Would you settle for a food that was 99.5 per cent artificial colouring-free?

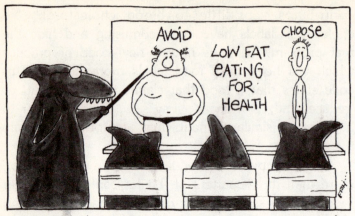

WHY THE INCIDENCE OF SHARK ATTACKS HAS FALLEN.

Codes of practice aren't perfect and some groups lobby successfully for exemptions. Margarines that are monounsaturated or polyunsaturated will still, unfortunately for waist-watchers, be able to carry a 'no cholesterol' tag even though such products still contain a substantial amount of saturated fat that can encourage the body to make cholesterol. The 'no cholesterol' claim on a margarine will also continue to confuse those people who think that 'no cholesterol' means 'no fat'. Margarines are 80 per cent fat, 'no cholesterol' or not.

Until the new code of practice is widely adopted, we will have a couple of years 'grace' for food manufacturers to make changes, so it will still pay to read the fine print carefully.

By law, labels must list ingredients in the order in which they come by weight in the product. The most prominent ingredient comes first, then the next and so on. If any kind of fat (such as those listed in the table below) comes in the first two or three ingredients in the list, beware!

Remember too, that *vegetable oil* or *vegetable fat* is **not** a guarantee that the fat is unsaturated. Vegetable fats and oils also have just as many calories as animal fats. Some food labels list *animal/vegetable fat*. This may mean that one or the other type of fat is used with the exact proportions depending on availability (or price). For the waist watcher, there's no difference in calories whichever type is used. For good health, there's also not much difference since most of the vegetable fats used in such products will have been **hydrogenated** (saturated) and will often contain at least as much, if not more, saturated fat as animal fat.

Foods sold in some countries must list the quantity of calories and certain nutrients. This is not yet required in Australia, except on foods that make any kind of nutritional claim. Once the product claims to be low in fat or salt, or high in calcium or fibre, or tells you of some other nutritional characteristic, the label must list the protein, fat, carbohydrate, kilojoules or calories, sodium and potassium. It must also disclose the amount of any other nutrient for which a claim is made.

Other names for fats in foods

vegetable oil/fat	animal fat/oil	shortening
tallow	coconut oil	palm oil
lard	chocolate	diglycerides
butter fat	milk solids	monoglycerides
copha	butter fat	chocolate chips

('creamed' and 'toasted' may also mean added fat)

GB high energy tip

*Avoid foods that have more than 10 g of fat per 100 g,
or that have fats as one of the first three ingredients.*
Become a 'fat detective' by checking all ingredient labels
for fat content.

You also need to know something about the com-
position of foods, especially when you are comparing
two foods, neither of which may be ideal. For example,
a low-fat spread for bread may be 50 or 60 per cent
fat. Although that is better than the 80 per cent fat
found in margarine and butter, it's still a lot. Even if
you only used 10 g of fat-reduced spread on each slice
of bread, you're still going to get 5 or 6 g of fat (instead
of 8 g from regular spreads).

By contrast, a turkey ham which is 97 per cent
fat-free (or a maximum of 3 per cent fat) is quite low

Table 6.1   *Deciphering an ingredient label:
nutrition information for a 100 g pack
of 'Lites' Potato Crisps*

	Per serving (50 g)	Per 100 g
Energy (Calories)	263	526
Protein	3.4 g	6.7 g
Fat	16.8 g	33.5 g
Carbohydrates		
total	26.8 g	53.5 g
sugars	0.2 g	0.3 g
Dietary fibre	2.7 g	5.4 g
Cholesterol	Negligible	Negligible
Sodium	295 mg	590 mg
Potassium	600 mg	1200 mg

in fat, especially if you use 50 g on a sandwich (in which case, you'll get less than 2 g of fat in a thick slice of sandwich filling).

The percentage of calories from fat is also used on some products. This is utterly confusing because it tells you nothing about how much fat you are actually getting. Many people also get confused between the percentage of fat in a product and the amount of energy (calories, kilojoules) derived from the fat.

For example, fish fillets may have only 2 per cent fat (that is, 2 g of fat in every 100 g of fish) but 16 per cent of its energy value (kilojoules) comes from fat. The first figure sounds quite moderate whereas the second sounds high. Fish is actually low in fat but because it's also low in calories, even a small amount of fat represents a high percentage. We can calculate it as follows: 100 g of fish has 2 g of fat and 28 g of protein. The 2 g of fat contribute 18 Calories (76 kJ) (9 Calories (38 kJ) from each gram); the 28 g of protein contribute 112 Calories (470 kJ) (4 Calories (17kJ) from each gram). Fish contains no carbohydrate so the total Calories from 100 g is 130 (18 + 112) (546 kJ). The percentage of calories from fat = 18/112 x 100 which is 16 per cent.

The percentage of calories coming from fat is only relevant at the end of the day when you add up all the

---

GB high energy tip

Don't drink alcohol and eat fatty foods (chips, peanuts etc.) together. Research shows that fat is stored more readily as fat if accompanied by alcohol.

fat and calories you have consumed and determine the total ratio. This is still fairly useless as it happens *after* the event—you've already eaten the food. It is not very informative for individual foods, as our fish example above shows.

The best way to count fat is to look at the grams of fat in a product and the total amount of fat that you're eating. For waist reduction, men should usually keep their total fat consumption below 40 g a day. You can tot up how much you're having during the day and stop choosing fat-containing foods when you reach your limit. It also helps to know which foods have little or no fat so that you can fill up on them.

If foods don't have the *amount* of fat per serving on the label but tell you their *percentage* of fat, try to choose those with less than 10 per cent fat.

The word *lite*, or some similar term on a food label, has also been misleading. *Lite* olive oil, for example, is light on flavour but has the same calorie level as any other olive oil. *Lite* crisps may be lightly salted but have the same number of calories as other crisps. *Lite* cheeses may have less fat than the regular products but their fat content may still be as high as 25 per cent of the product weight (regular cheese has 33 per cent fat by weight).

To summarise our simple recommendations about fat in foods:

- Try to keep below a daily total of 40 g of fat.
- Avoid foods with more than 10 per cent fat (or more than 10 g per 100 g. That is, go only for those marked 90 per cent fat-free or more. (*Note*: not '90 per cent less fat' as this only means less than it was before.)

The new code of practice says that manufacturers must tell you which characteristic of a food makes it *lite* or *light*. For example, a potato crisp or olive oil that is 'light in flavour' must say so. The packet cannot simply be labelled *light*.

Thin potato crisps may also sound appealing to those watching their waistline but these are not low in calories. With any food fried in oil or fat, the greater the surface area, the greater the uptake of oil or fat. Thin crisps or small potato chips will usually have a higher fat and calorie level than fatter (as in thicker) products. A potato has no fat and only 70 Calories (294 kJ) per 100 g. Homemade thick potato chips have 190 Calories (798 kJ) per 100 g. Crinkle cut potato chips have 290 Calories (1218 kJ) per 100 g. Fine cut chips have 365 Calories (1533 kJ) per 100 g. Potato crisps, the thinnest of them all, have 525 Calories (2205 kJ) per 100 g. (You might like to compare the price you're paying for potatoes. The smaller the piece, the higher the price— and the higher the fat content.)

To help further, where a claim about a food would apply to the whole class of foods, the label must say so. For example, brand X baked beans that claim the product is high in fibre will have to say *baked beans are high in fibre*, without implying that it is just their brand that has lots of fibre.

Making good choices

Some foods are inherently fatty. But sometimes better choices can be made. Check out the table below before choosing.

Which is better—butter or margarine?

We must point out that butter and margarine have the same high fat content—80 g in every 100 g. Butter fell from favour in the 1970s because it has a high content of saturated fat. Margarine moved in to take over the yellow spread market and those labelled *poly-unsaturated* were perceived as healthier because they helped lower blood cholesterol levels.

In the 1990s, polyunsaturated margarine has fallen from its perch. In large quantities, polyunsaturated fats can lower beneficial HDL cholesterol levels. They also oxidise more rapidly and contribute to the formation of nasty plaque in the walls of arteries, unless more foods rich in antioxidants (fruits, vegetables, red wine, some grains and legumes, tea) are consumed. Marga-

Table 6.2

Food	Fat content (g)	Less fatty choice	Fat content (g)
Butter, 1 tbsp	16	Reduced-fat butter, 1 tbsp	10
Margarine, 1 tbsp	16	Reduced-fat margarine, 1 tbsp	8
Cheddar cheese, 50 g	16	Fat-reduced cheese, 50 g	12
Regular milk, 250mL	10	Fat-reduced milk, 250mL	3–4
Fat-reduced milk, 250 mL	3–4	Skim milk or Shape, 250 mL	0
Cream, 2 tbsp	7	Lite cream, 2 tbsp	3
French dressing, 2 tbsp	10	No oil French dressing, 2 tbsp	0
Mayonnaise, 1 tbsp	7	Lite mayonnaise, 1 tbsp	2
Regular sausages, 2	32	Lite sausages, 2	6

rines also contain an undesirable type of trans fatty acids. The final nail was hammered into the margarine coffin when a major study of over 89 000 nurses found that those who ate the most margarine had the most heart disease.

Manufacturers are now making mono-unsaturated margarines because this type of fat doesn't oxidise as rapidly. Unfortunately, most of these products still contain trans fatty acids.

Conclusion: neither butter or margarine is very desirable. The less yellow spreads waist watchers eat, the better.

Hydrogenation

This processing method turns a liquid oil into a spreadable product by converting some of the unsaturated fats into saturated ones. Trans fatty acids are also formed— generally making up about 12 per cent of margarines, as we have mentioned.

Hydrogenation is also used in making fats for pastries, biscuits and other bakery products. Some of these products can have a high content of trans fatty acids.

Conclusion: avoid eating too many hydrogenated fats. Read labels. They won't *always* tell you about the presence of hydrogenisation, but they often will.

GB high energy tip

Rinse hamburger meat to reduce fat. Par cook hamburger mince, drain the fat, then rinse with warm water before completely cooking. This can reduce fat content by 20–30 per cent.

7 Fibre, flatulence and fatness

One of the key recommendations of the GutBuster Program is to eat more fibre. Fibre and fatness don't seem to go together, probably because fibre is so filling. But here's a warning: fibre and flatulence *do* go together. You may find that reducing fat in your diet gives you a feeling of jumping over the moon, but the extra fibre provides its own activity!

You may have trouble convincing the females in your life, but there's good news attached to wind. While helpful bacteria in your bowel are busy producing gases, they also produce some valuable acids that can help reduce your risk of bowel cancer.

Be assured that wind is normal.
Even your mother has it.

It's normal to produce gases and Professor Terry

70

Bolin and Rosemary Stanton found that the average male lets fly about 13 times a day while the average woman bottom burps about seven or eight times. Those who eat more fibre pass wind more often—up to twenty times a day is quite common—and it's normal and healthy. Bolin and Stanton's book, *Wind Breaks* (Margaret Gee, 1993), will answer everything you always wanted to know about flatulence but were too embarrassed to ask. Be assured, however, that wind is normal—even your mother has it! It may be a social problem but it's not usually a medical one. If the embarrassment is too great, there are ways to ease you into a less windy environment, as we'll see in this chapter.

What is fibre anyway?

In spite of its name, dietary fibre is not always fibrous. The scientific term for dietary fibre is *non-starch poly-saccharide*. The *saccharide* part of the term gives away the fact that dietary fibre is related to carbohydrate. In layman's language, dietary fibre comprises those parts of plant foods that resist digestion in the small intestine (where almost all the other digestion occurs) and pass through to the large intestine (also called the *large bowel* or *colon*). Most types of fibre are attacked and digested by good and helpful bacteria in the large bowel. As the bacteria are breaking down the fibre, they get enough energy to multiply furiously. Bacteria don't have a long life and when they've finished it, their dead bodies form a large part of what we excrete. One type of fibre called lignin is too much even for the staunchest bacteria. Nothing can attack it and it passes out intact. The spent bodies of the bacteria, plus lignin and water make up the bulk of what we excrete.

Dietary fibre exists in two main classes: soluble and insoluble. Soluble fibre includes pectins (in fruits), hemi-celluloses (in fruits, vegetables, legumes, some cereals) and gums and mucilages (in some fruits, seeds and legumes). Soluble fibres are completely broken down by bacteria and contribute to the bulk of faeces by increasing the number of bacteria (whose dead bodies then contribute bulk). Insoluble fibres include cellulose (in fruits, vegetables, wholegrain cereals) and lignin (in cereal husks or brans and in some fruits and vegetables). Some cellulose is broken down by bacteria (to a greater extent in women than in men) but lignin escapes untouched.

Is soluble or insoluble fibre better? Neither type of fibre is *better* than the other. Both are useful and serve different purposes. Soluble fibre is useful in the stomach and small intestine because it slows down the rate of digestion in this part of the gut, so you feel full for longer. Insoluble fibre gives a greater feeling of fullness lower down within the gut. So both types of fibre create feelings of fullness.

Some people think that fibre passes straight through

GB high energy tip

Eat 3–4 pieces of different fruit and 4–5 vegetables every day. Fruit and vegetables are high in fibre and filling. Where feasible eat the skins as well, as these are even higher in fibre.

the gut and that means you don't absorb any calories from high-fibre foods. That's too simplistic. We get fewer calories from fibre than from anything else we eat because the bacteria use up some of them. Researchers still debate how many calories high-fibre foods give us, but most agree it's only 2–3 Calories (8–12 kJ) per gram of dietary fibre. Lignin doesn't contribute any calories because it isn't broken down at all.

Why all the talk about fibre?

The importance of fibre has been known for centuries. Aristotle preached its virtues but then, like many things, it was forgotten for many years. Occasionally it reared its head. Dr Allinson wrote an essay in the 1880s linking a lack of fibre with haemorrhoids (piles), constipation and varicose veins. Allinson's high-fibre bread recipe is still made in Britain and in some parts of Australia. During World War II, a surgeon called (no kidding) Captain Cleave, noted that a lack of fibre made sailors constipated, decreased size of stools and increased the time food took to pass through the gut. He fed them bran, banned sugar and alerted the Western world to the fact that its diet was not perfect.

In the 1960s Dr Denis Burkitt, a surgeon who had worked in East Africa for twenty years, succeeded in bringing the world's attention back to fibre. Burkitt and his co-workers noticed that Africans eating a diet very high in plant foods did not suffer from many common Western diseases. Burkitt armed himself with a bucket and spade and followed Bantu bushmen gathering proof of his theory that small stools led to the need for large hospitals. Rural Africans produced stools like a reversed spinning top—flat surface down and pointed on top— with usual daily stool weight around 400–500 g. Westerners, by contrast, tend to produce 'balls, buttons or bullets'—daily weight 80 to 120 g. The intestinal transit time (that is, the time taken for food residues to pass from the mouth to the anus) is about one and a half days in rural Africans and twice as long in Westerners.

Burkitt decided that these differences had nothing to do with the climate or racial characteristics but had everything to do with diet. Having noted that bowel cancer, appendicitis, diverticular disease and various other gut problems were common in Westerners and almost non-existent in rural Africans, Burkitt put two and two together and came up with the fibre theory. Fibre is good for you, he said, and we should all eat more of it. He included some brief references to obesity being more

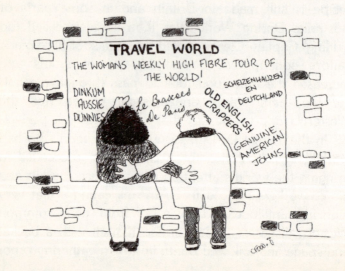

common in those who ate little fibre but the real evidence linking a lot of fibre with less fat came later.

The next stage was predictable. Food manufacturers decided to stop throwing away the bran fibre they were stripping from wheat and sell it separately. Pharmaceutical companies decided to compress it into tablets and then moved on to making various other fibre supplements from the left-over fibres from refined food. This is obviously quite absurd. We start with a good whole food, refine and process it and then sell people back some of the bits. What's wrong with eating the whole food in the first place? The answer is simple. Separating food into parts and re-selling various sections brings in better profits. It may not, however, give the consumer all the advantages of eating the whole food. Unprocessed wheat bran is a good example. Whole-wheat or wholemeal products should contain the whole grain. Turning wheat into white flour and then convincing people to eat the rather unpalatable bran doesn't have the same benefits. Too much separated unprocessed bran can even be harmful, decreasing absorption of some minerals and damaging cells in the bowel.

There's more to fibre than bran, just as there's more to fruit than vitamin C and more to fish than you'll get from fish oil capsules. You can't beat whole food for good nutritional value and high-fibre foods are no exception.

Foods high in fibre

Fruits These are good sources of fibre. Some fibre is found in the skin so it's silly to waste it if it's edible.

Some gummy types of fibre are found close to the skin. All fruits have fibre but the richest sources are raspberries and blackberries, passionfruit, prunes, dried apricots, pears, bananas, oranges and apples.

Vegetables These provide lots of fibre, especially peas, spinach, artichokes, broccoli, Brussels sprouts, carrots and pumpkin. Even the good old spud is a good source of fibre. It is not one of the richest sources, but eating potatoes regularly makes them a good standard base.

Legumes Chick peas, lentils and various types of beans (including canned beans) are the best sources of fibre of all. These foods are so rich in fibre, especially soluble fibre, that eating them at lunch means that you are unlikely to start picking in the afternoon. But legumes do give you extra wind. (Bolin and Stanton's book *Wind Breaks* gives some clues for reducing gas production from beans.)

Bread This is a good source of fibre. Wholemeal or wholegrain breads have the highest fibre content, followed by multigrain, rye breads, fibre-increased white loaves and, bottom of the class, white bread. However, even though white bread has less fibre than wholemeal, it is still a good food which is low in fat, high in complex carbohydrate and with more than enough vitamins. For waist-watchers who feel hungry easily, go for wholemeal or wholegrain breads for first preference in breads. If they're not available, have any kind of bread that appeals to you.

Breakfast cereals These are a mixed bag when it comes to dietary fibre. Some have lots while others

---

GB high energy tip

Eat 6–8 slices of (wholemeal or wholegrain) bread a day. Bread is a good source of fibre and is low in fat. It's the spreads put on bread, not the bread itself, which are fattening.

---

have very little. Bran-based cereals are high in fibre. Wholewheat, oat or barley-based products are also good sources of fibre. Unprocessed wheat bran is high in fibre but you need to take care to choose a brand that has not been too finely milled. Big flakes of unprocessed bran absorb water in the bowel and give bulk to stools. Finely milled bran absorbs less water, forms pellets and can increase constipation. Highly-processed cereals such as cornflakes and rice bubbles have little or no fibre.

Grains Rice, wheat, rye, millet, buckwheat (not strictly a grain), oats and barley, and foods made from them such as cracked wheat (bulgur) and pasta, are good sources of fibre. Wholegrain or wholemeal versions such as brown rice or wholemeal pasta have the most fibre. If you don't like wholemeal pasta, it's good to know that even the regular types are a good source of fibre.

Nuts and seeds These also supply dietary fibre. In small quantities they cause no problems, but if once you start eating nuts you find it difficult to stop, you can easily blow your fat intake for the day.

'Resistant' starch

Some starches are not degraded by the usual enzymes in the small intestine and pass to the large bowel (colon) where they are fermented by bacteria, just as dietary fibre is. Bananas, rice cooked by the absorption method (with just enough water so that it's all taken up by the rice), potatoes cooked and then cooled, and some other foods contain resistant starch.

Medical researchers now believe that resistant starch may be even more important than dietary fibre because it can be present in much larger amounts than fibre.

The wind in the pillows

When fibre and resistant starch are broken down by bacteria in the bowel, valuable acids and some gases are produced. The acids are good for you, keeping bowel cells healthy and resistant to bowel cancer and helping to stimulate the muscular action that moves food wastes along the length of the intestine. The gases are a by-product and they have to be released. The closest exit is what you're sitting on. The gases include hydrogen, oxygen, nitrogen, sulphur and, in some people, methane. We don't know why some people produce methane and others don't. Nor do we know if it's good to produce methane or not. You may or may not produce methane, but everyone produces the other gases. Some people produce more than others and eating more fibre will increase gas production in everyone. This may be socially embarrassing but it's quite healthy and, unless it's really excessive or accompanied by pain, gas is not a medical problem. At some stage, gas needs to come out, although it doesn't hurt to hold on to it for a short while. Babies and the elderly may have less elasticity in the bowel and may find it more difficult to hold on to it. Babies generally don't even try!

More gas is produced after meals and this depends to some extent on the type of foods eaten. This subject is going to get just a little bit worse before we finish, so here goes. Most people worry not so much about producing gas but about the *aroma* it has. High-fibre eaters can relax at this point because although fibre increases the *amount* of gas produced, it's not fibre itself that causes the odour. A high-protein diet, especially one containing a lot of meat, and spices are the main contributors to aromatic flatus. Beans may cause some increase in odour, probably because they are high in protein as well as fibre.

Those who suffer from excessive gas, or who have any diarrhoea, bloating or pain associated with it, should see their doctor. The most common reason is an intolerance to lactose (the sugar present naturally in milk), but you shouldn't assume that this is the basis of your problems. Doctors can do special tests to diagnose lactose intolerance. In the meantime, there are some other methods of reducing excessive flatulence outlined by Bolin and Stanton and summarised in the table below.

Fibre and bowel motions

If you eat more fibre, you will probably find a change in your daily toilet practices. More fibre increases both

Table 7.1 Likely causes and possible cures for flatulence

Cause	Possible cure
Legumes (dried beans, peas)	Increase consumption gradually
	Soak overnight, pour off soaking water (add 1/2 teaspoon mustard seeds to soaking water)
Cauliflower, broccoli, Brussels sprouts	Reduce cooking time
Unripe fruits	Wait until they ripen
Fruit juices	Avoid, especially apple and pear juice
Fatty foods	Decrease
Milk	Substitute calcium-enriched soy (low fat)*

* Check with doctor that lactose is the problem. Small quantities of milk (up to half a cup), yoghurt and cheese should not cause problems.

stool frequency and quantity. High-fibre stools also float more because they contain more air. This is normal and is no cause for concern. It may sound like a morbid activity to take note of what comes and goes from your body, but a bit less coyness about such subjects would help reduce the high incidence of bowel cancer. If you notice any blood in your stools or on the toilet paper, or if you have had a close family relative with bowel cancer, you need to see your doctor, especially if you're over 40. The most common cause of blood on the toilet paper is haemorrhoids (piles) but this can sometimes be a smokescreen. Small growths called polyps can be growing in the bowel and these may also be contributing to the blood you see. A special test called a colonoscopy can find and remove polyps before they become cancerous. Bowel cancer is the most common internal cancer in Australia. It's treatable—if caught early.

GB high energy tip

Keep your eye on the bowel. With an increase in fibre in the diet, daily motions may increase in frequency, size and colour and tend to float more. Check with your doctor if any blood is present.

Summary
The main advantages of dietary fibre are:
- It's bulky and slows down the rate at which the stomach empties so that you feel full for longer (especially true of soluble fibre).
- It tends to decrease the appetite for fatty foods.
- It keeps the bowel healthy and reduces the chance of constipation, haemorrhoids and bowel cancer.
- Foods high in fibre are also rich in vitamins, minerals and antioxidants.
- High-fibre foods taste good.
- A high-fibre diet will change your bowel habits and probably increase flatulence, but this should be less odorous than on a high protein diet.

8 Sugar: how sweet it isn't!

The major nutritional thrust of the GutBuster Program has been to decrease fat and increase dietary fibre. We've praised high-fibre carbohydrate-rich foods such as breads, cereals, grains and fruit. Sugar is also a carbohydrate food so we need to come up with some explanations about how sugar should fit in to your eating patterns. Do we mean that you should fill up on sugar as well?

The answer is NO. Sugar is not a filling food like the other carbohydrate foods we've been praising. It's certainly not as bad as fat, as we've already pointed out, but sugar doesn't fill you up either. And it certainly doesn't take away your appetite—if anything, it's likely to stimulate it. You can add sugar to water, as in soft drinks or cordials, and it won't fill you up any more than plain water. Sweet drinks don't even quench your thirst as well as plain water, so they often encourage you to take in even more sugars. So we suggest that decreasing sugars—at least to some extent—will add the icing to (or perhaps, remove it from) the cake of your high energy program.

Of course, simply cutting back on fat removes a lot of sugar from the diet. If you've switched to bread, pasta, rice, fruit and beans instead of eating lots of pastries, pies, cakes, biscuits, chocolate and fatty desserts, you'll already have reduced the amount of sugar you eat. Sugar makes fat taste nice and the company sugar often keeps is one of its worst features.

Carbohydrates—simple and complex

Carbohydrates are organic compounds containing carbon, oxygen and hydrogen. The ratio of hydrogen to oxygen is 2:1, as in water, so that a carbohydrate is really a 'hydrate of carbon'.

Most carbohydrates come from plant sources, although there are exceptions, such as lactose, the sugar found in the milk of all mammals, and ribose, which is made within the body as part of the overall energy system. Many carbohydrates in plants are made by the process of photosynthesis, using carbon dioxide and water with energy from sunlight. Carbohydrates are thus basic building blocks which trap energy and give life to the animal kingdom.

Carbohydrates include sugars, starches, glycogen (in liver and muscles), dextrins (gummy forms of starch) and dietary fibre. The simplest classification is to divide the carbohydrates into simple sugars and complex carbohydrates, also called starches. After digestion in the human intestine, all carbohydrates are broken down to simple sugars to be used to produce energy. Carbohydrates can therefore be considered *energy foods*.

Most people are aware of the sugar industry promotions that tell us that sugar is a *natural part of life*. It wasn't always so, and the white sugar crystals that have invaded the food supply over the past century have not been a major part of life throughout human history. Refined sugar is a relatively recent product. Sugar was first produced around 500 BC by boiling down the juice pressed from sugar cane and allowing the liquid to evaporate to produce dark brown crystals. Some 700 years later, small amounts of sugar were being produced in North Africa, Spain and Syria but it wasn't until the Spanish introduced sugar cane to the Caribbean in the sixteenth century that the potential for sugar production was realised. Even then, it was not until slaves were brought from Africa to carry out the physically demanding job of growing and cutting cane in a hot climate that sugar consumption really took off.

The average person now consumes the equivalent of 230 cubes of sugar each week in food and drinks.

Sugar's history is not pretty and it is somewhat ironic that it should taste so sweet when its production brought so much blood, sweat and tears to so many people. To add to its bad reputation, sugar lacks any vestige of protein, vitamin, mineral, essential fatty acid or fibre. In spite of this, the average person now consumes the equivalent of 230 cubes of sugar each week in food and drinks. When you consider that some people don't get through their share, it means that others really take in a lot. Even the average consumption contributes 500 Calories (2100 kJ) a day, quite a significant amount for waist control.

Most people think of sugar as being fattening and most weight control programs cut out sugar. Some of the more foolish programs restrict all carbohydrates, trying to achieve maximum *weight* loss through the loss of water associated with a low-carbohydrate intake. Unfortunately, with very little energy-giving carbohydrate, you become tired, irritable and find exercise difficult. Few people can stick to such diets for long.

In general, we know that the body does not turn complex carbohydrate into fat until the level is high— equivalent to the amount in about 35 slices of bread. The GutBuster Program has therefore worked on the principle of freely allowing carbohydrates but restricting fats (which are easily turned into body fat). We've always favoured carbohydrates that are also rich in dietary fibre such as bread, cereals and wholegrain foods, potatoes, peas, beans and fruit because they're filling. We've not been really strict about sugar, because the level of sugar is automatically reduced when you restrict fats (many fatty foods are sweet).

GB high energy tip

Don't eat fatty and sugary foods together at the same meal. Recent research shows that fat may be stored more readily in the presence of sugar, so avoid a fatty main course followed by sweets.

The GutBuster Program aims to keep metabolism high so that more calories (from food and body fat) are burned. You can't ignore the fact that a body that is amply supplied with calories from a food such as sugar will not need to use up its own fat supplies. Since the GutBuster Program supplies plenty of other, more nutritious carbohydrate foods, sugar is not needed as an energy source. Until we understand more about the way in which the body converts sugar into fat, it makes sense for waist-watchers to go easy on sugar because insulin resistance may make it less likely that sugar's energy will be burned as fuel.

Classifying carbohydrates

We classify carbohydrates according to their molecular structure, in a similar way to fats.

Sugars

Monosaccharides These are simple sugars made up of five or six carbon atoms (usually six). They're called *mono* because they have a single unit that represents the smallest type of sugar molecule. The three main monosaccharides are:

1 *glucose*—found in fruits, vegetables and honey
2 *fructose*—found in honey and fruits
3 *galactose*—found only in very small quantities in fruits and vegetables and formed mainly from the breakdown of lactose, the sugar in milk.

All the monosaccharides taste sweet. Fructose is the sweetest. Ribose is a five-carbon monosaccharide formed in the body and used in the cycle that produces energy as fuel.

Disaccharides These are *double* sugars with two monosaccharides joined together. They're broken down in the small intestine into their two component monosaccharides. The most commonly occurring disaccharides are:

1 *Sucrose*. Found mainly in sugar cane, but also in some fruits and vegetables, it comprises one molecule of glucose and one of fructose.
2 *Lactose*. Found only in the milk of mammals, including human milk, it comprises one molecule of glucose and one of galactose.
3 *Maltose*. Found in sprouting wheat and in malted grains, it comprises two molecules of glucose.

Oligosaccharides Also known as *dextrins*, these molecules have 3 to 15 monosaccharides linked in a chain. They are formed when starches are being digested.

Complex carbohydrates

Once known as polysaccharides, these carbohydrates have either straight or branched chains of monosaccharides which may be all the same type or different types. They include starches, glycogen (storage starch found in muscles and liver), cellulose, gums and other types of dietary fibre. These are larger molecules and usually take longer to be broken down to glucose than simple sugars. They provide a slower, more sustained release of energy.

Which carbo?

As we've seen, complex carbohydrate foods are unlikely to cause any problems. They are both filling and wholesome foods. It is really only refined sugar foods that needed to be avoided in a waist control or a high energy program. These occur when the basic sugar has been stripped from its parent food, making over-consumption possible and easy. For example, you couldn't chew your way through the amount of sugar cane needed to produce the average consumption of sugar but it's not difficult to get through a large amount when it's dissolved in drinks, syrups or added to sweet and fatty foods. Similarly, it would take a long time to munch your way through four or five apples but only seconds to down the sugar once it's been refined as fruit juice.

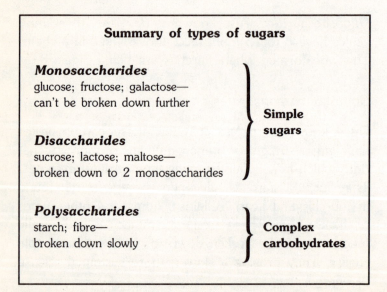

Summary of types of sugars

Monosaccharides
glucose; fructose; galactose—
can't be broken down further

⎫
⎬ **Simple**
⎭ **sugars**

Disaccharides
sucrose; lactose; maltose—
broken down to 2 monosaccharides

Polysaccharides
starch; fibre—
broken down slowly

⎫
⎬ **Complex**
⎭ **carbohydrates**

GB high energy tip

Don't drink anything you can eat whole. Avoid fruit juices, but eat the whole fruit instead. It has fewer calories, more fibre and is more filling.

Recognising sugar

Everyone recognises the white crystals that make up regular cane sugar. A level measuring teaspoon of sugar weighing 4 grams has 16 calories. A typical sugar-spoonful has twice as many. Even taking one sugar in half a dozen cups of tea and coffee a day can add up to almost 200 Calories, so it's worth gradually training your tastebuds to like unsweetened beverages, or use artificial sweeteners.

Replacing white sugar with brown sugar, honey, raw sugar, glucose or castor sugar has no effect because they're all sugars with the same energy density. There are also sugars which are less easily recognisable or sound even more favourable. Some of these are shown in the box below:

Other names for sugars on ingredient labels

- glucose
- lactose
- cane sugar
- beet sugar
- treacle
- dextrose
- raw sugar
- demerara sugar
- honey
- sorbitol
- maltose
- brown sugar
- maple sugar
- molasses

As more than 80 per cent of the sugar we consume comes from processed foods and drinks, it's worth knowing where it comes from. You might expect to find sugar in jam, sweetened canned fruit, cordials, syrups and soft drinks but it's also in less commonly expected places like peanut butter, chicken soup, baked beans, tomato sauce, canned vegetables, cracker biscuits and hamburger buns. It's also used to sweeten medicine and makes up much of the weight of many vitamin tablets and cough lollies.

Remember that ingredients must be listed on labels in their order of *prominence* in a product. If the total sugar content is high and sugar would therefore be the first ingredient, some manufacturers get around the problem by using several different sugars. For example, if you were making an apricot *health* bar with 40 per cent apricots and 60 per cent sugar, you would have to list the ingredients as *sugar, apricots*. If you use 20 per cent each of three different sugars, the ingredients could be listed as *apricots, raw sugar, honey, fructose*. You should always read labels and count the number of different types of sugar in the first part of the ingredient list. If sugars occur frequently, you can probably bet that the total sugar content is high. You've probably noticed sugars' names often end in the letters *-ose* so this is one thing to look out for.

How much sugar?

You don't need to avoid all sugar but you should be aware of its presence and the contribution that sugars of all types make to calorie intake.

We talked about either trying to keep total fat intake below about 40 grams per day, or to choose foods with less than 10 per cent fat. With sugar, it makes

---

GB high energy tip

Avoid foods with several forms of sugar high on the ingredient list. To hide the amount of sugar used, manufacturers often split 'sugar' into its constituent sugars so that these can be put lower down on the ingredient list.

---

sense to keep below a daily total of 20 to 25 grams. It can be difficult to add this up because most food labels group together the sugars occurring in ingredients such as fruits with the added sugar. A practical suggestion is to try to avoid foods whose labels state they have more than 10 grams of added simple sugars per serve. This method doesn't work for foods that contain dried fruit, as the naturally occurring sugar in these foods may increase the sugars listed on the label. The sugar in fruit and dried fruit is not considered a problem as it comes with valuable dietary fibre, vitamins and minerals. However, eating large quantities of dried fruit will slow down waist loss.

The digestion of sugars and starches

There is no digestion of sugars until they reach the small intestine. Here they are broken down into monosaccharides. Those that are already in this form do not need further breakdown.

The digestion of complex carbohydrate (starch) begins in the mouth where an enzyme present in saliva starts breaking the polysaccharides into smaller units. This is one reason why it is so important to chew food properly. Once the complex carbohydrate is swallowed the acid which is normally found in the stomach stops this action and the starch must then wait until it reaches the small intestine for the enzymes there to complete the process.

Contrary to popular belief, there's no need to eat sugars and starches on their own. It's quite normal for food to wait in the stomach for a while before entering the small intestine for its major digestion. If this does not occur, and the food passes quickly into the small intestine, you feel hungry quickly. Try eating some fruit on an empty stomach to experience this. If you have some cereal with your fruit, it slows the emptying of the stomach so you don't feel hungry quite so quickly. This is an advantage and those who espouse the wonders of *food combining* (which usually means *not* combining certain foods) know little about human nutrition. Fruit eaten with other foods does *not* rot and ferment in the stomach as some people believe.

After sugar is broken down into its component monosaccharides, these are absorbed from the small intestine into the bloodstream. The presence of sugars in the blood triggers the pancreas to release insulin, a hormone that helps sugars pass from the blood into the cells to be used as an energy source. Insulin thus has a *gatekeeper* role. With some simple sugars, so much may enter the bloodstream so quickly that there may be an insulin overshoot. If there is any insulin resistance (because of a build-up of fat within the membrane around the cell), the sugar does not enter the cell and is more likely to be converted to body fat. The old idea of taking something sweet as an energy boost, for example before sport, is not valid, especially if there is an insulin overshoot. In fact, this can cause a *decrease* in energy 20 to 30 minutes later.

Energy within muscles is present as glycogen. It takes many hours (often as much as 24 hours) for any type of carbohydrate to form glycogen in muscles, so nothing eaten immediately before sport will contribute to this type of muscle energy. For those wanting a pre-game booster, it's best to have some complex carbohydrate a couple of hours before. It will be broken down and ready as blood sugar by the time you're set to go. However we can't be exact about this, because the rates at which sugars enter the bloodstream depend on what else you have eaten. Fats, for example, will slow down the emptying of the stomach. To boost muscle glycogen supplies, you need to eat more carbohydrate 24 hours before exercise.

It is important for sports people to take note of replenishing carbohydrate *after* a bout of heavy exercise. This is one time when a simple carbohydrate is preferable, as we know that muscles that have just been depleted of their glycogen supplies will make more

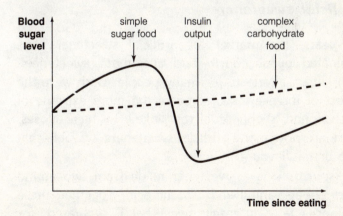

Digestion of carbohydrates

GB high energy tip

Avoid foods with more than 10 grams of simple sugars per serving size. Many foods now have low calorie alternatives. Check the sugar content and serving size.

---

glycogen in a much shorter time if there is some rapidly-absorbed carbohydrate coming into the body within the first 30 minutes after physical activity. Complex carbohydrates will be broken down and absorbed too slowly to be of much use in this situation. They are important as follow-on carbohydrates once the immediate need for rapidly-absorbed carbohydrates has been met. This is really only important for those who do very strenuous activity every day. (For more information, see Rosemary Stanton's *Eating for Peak Performance,* 2nd edition, Allen & Unwin, Sydney, 1994.)

Artificial sweeteners

For years, the market for artificial sweeteners was dominated by *saccharin* and *cyclamate* sweeteners. Both left an aftertaste for many people. Both were the subject of intense tests, some of the more extreme of which found slight problems linked to huge doses. There are now many artificial sweeteners available that have better flavour.

Aspartame is a sweetener made from two amino acids, phenylalanine and aspartic acid. Together, these substances taste intensely sweet but if separated, for example in cooking, they no longer taste sweet.

Aspartame is sold as Equal and is available either in tablets or a sprinkle-on table-top form.

Slenda is a sweetener made from sugar but with chlorine atoms replacing some of the normal atoms on the sucrose molecule. It has the advantage of being stable to heat and can be used in baking. It is used in some yoghurt products and is available for home use.

Acesulfame K (the *K* is for potassium) is another intense sweetener used in some processed foods.

Other sweeteners are also appearing on the market. Each is a substance that tastes intensely sweet so that only very small quantities are needed, compared with sugar. This means that they contribute virtually no calories. Before being released, they are subject to stringent testing. If sugar was tested in the same way, it would probably fail.

There is little doubt that sweeteners are safe in the quantities usually consumed. Any harmful effects are at levels that would be impossible to achieve. Almost any food given in very high doses will produce symptoms in some people. Artificial sweeteners seem to be no exception. Just as anyone who experiences symptoms after eating bananas or tomatoes should avoid those foods, so anyone who gets headaches or other problems after sweeteners should avoid them. Tests show

---

GB high energy tip

Use an artificial sweetener instead of sugar if you can't do without the taste of sweetness. It may take a week or two to adapt to the taste of sweeteners, but these are low calorie and safe.

that the chances of anyone having any problems is extremely small and sweeteners can therefore be considered safe.

For those who love sweetness, these products can be useful. However, as long as you keep using such products, you are unlikely to allow your taste-buds to adjust to less sweetness. Artificial sweeteners, like fake fats, preserve a love of sweetness (or fat). Those who give up sweeteners (or fats) find that they don't like them as much after about three months. Many people try giving up sugar or fatty foods but don't persevere for long enough. From research into taste-bud response to salt, fat or sugar, we know that changes in palatability take time. But if you really want sweetness, use artificial sweeteners by all means. At least they don't contribute to dental decay, as sugar can so easily do and they also have virtually no calories.

III
Making the most of movement

9 Not exercise— movement!

The word 'exercise' is enough to frighten most people off—that is, at least the 85 per cent of individuals who don't do it regularly. So we try not to use the term in relation to fat loss. Instead, we talk about *movement*. Now there is a difference—a big difference—especially when it comes to the type of movement needed to get rid of *fat*, compared with that needed for getting *fit*.

If you look at most books and programs on exercise (even some of our own), it's exercise for fitness, not fatness, that is emphasised. And although the prescriptions for fitness are fairly standard, you'll probably be bamboozled by the way in which they are presented. Here is a typical quote:

'. . . exercise at a rate that is 60–80 per cent of maximum heart rate (which is 200 minus your age), aerobically for 30 minutes at least 3–4 days per week.'

Until recently it was thought that this was also the formula for reducing fatness. And this is one of the reasons why the fitness industry and the fatness industry are poles apart (how many fat people do you see in gyms?). We do know that fat is only oxidised, or 'burned up', at low levels of exercise intensity, when oxygen is being used—that is during *aerobic* exercise. When exercise becomes more intense, lactic acid, a by-product of the glucose used for fuel, accumulates in the muscles and inhibits fat oxidation. Intense exercise, where oxygen is not involved, is called *anaerobic* (without air) exercise. Here, the main fuel is glucose which can come from carbohydrate in food, blood glucose or a form of glucose stored in muscles and the liver called glycogen. Fat is not used as a fuel for anaerobic exercise. Doing anything too vigorous then— *busting* a gut—is not going to help you to *lose* a gut. All it does is help burn up those sugars, mainly from carbohydrates, that are in the bloodstream or stored in muscle or the liver.

There is a possible caveat to this however, which again highlights the advantages of being male (at least in relation to fat loss). Young men (that is, those less than 40 years of age) it seems will lose fat in response to just about any form of exercise. From an evolution-

---

GB high energy tip

To burn fat, slow down and go longer and more continuously. Fat as a fuel is only burned in the presence of oxygen (aerobically), and so optimal fat burning requires low speed and long duration.

ary point of view this is probably because men have been designed to cope with long periods of aerobic expenditure of energy in looking for game for food and short bursts of anaerobic energy expenditure chasing and catching it. Women, on the other hand, were designed to spend long aerobic periods gathering nuts, seeds, berries, yams and other vegetables. If a woman exercised hard (anaerobically), this probably spelt danger in a hunter–gatherer environment. For a woman, danger then means slowing down the rate of fat-burning to increase her chances of survival (through reserve fat stores) so the species could survive. This is now one reason proposed for why women tend to become resistant to fat loss under extreme exercise loads, whereas men shed it quite easily, almost irrespective of what type of exercise they do. But since we know that low intensity exercise is all that's needed, why bust a gut?

With improvements in exercise science it is now clear that there are many different forms of effective exercise training. The one you choose depends on your goals. Training for competitive sport, for example, is quite different from the kind of exercise required for general cardiovascular fitness. Training for muscle gain is different from that required for fat loss. Some of the differences between different efforts are shown in Table 9.1 below.

As you can see from this table, exercise for fitness, and therefore high energy gain, needs to be done at a vigorous level, over short periods, 3–4 days a week. Obviously, this is not ideal (and is likely to be dangerous) for anyone who has a low level of fitness or a

Table 9.1 Exercise parameters for different goals

	Competitive sport	Cardio-vascular fitness	Fatness	Muscle			Flexibility
				power	strength	bulk	
Frequency	2–3 times daily	3–4 days/week	6–7 days/week	Varies in season	Alternate days (most muscle groups)	Alternate days	Regularly
Intensity	Up to maximum	60–80% max.	40–60% max.	40–80% max.	Max.	60–80% max.	Very low
Time	Very long total time 3–5 hours	Relatively short 30 mins	Long 1+ hours	Short	Long	Long	Short–medium
Type	Sport related totally planned	Aerobic/anaerobic planned	Aerobic only (a) planned (b) incidental	Resistance	Resistance	Resistance	Stretching
Continuity	Intervals	Interval/continuous	Continuous		Intermittent		N/A
Speed	Generally fastest	Medium	Slow	Very fast	Slow–medium	Slow–medium	Very slow

high level of fatness. The best type of exercise for fat loss, on the other hand, is not 'exercise' at all, but movement—long, slow, continuous and often. And, as can be seen from Table 9.1, there are two main types: planned or organised movement, and incidental movement.

Planned (organised) movement

'Planned movement' means planning a low intensity activity for a set duration or distance, as often as possible. In the past, this wouldn't have been necessary. For around 99 570 of the past 100 000 years of evolution, humans have had enough movement in their day-to-day lives just to survive, that they had no chance to become obese. It's only during the last 30 years that machines and modern technology have taken over doing much of this for us and so it has become necessary to 'institutionalise' movement by setting aside a particular time of the day, and a place, to carry it out.

The simplest movement for most people is walking. In the first phase of the GutBuster Program, in contrast to many other weight control programs, we set a distance and not a time for planned movement. This is because with very unfit and overfat men, there is always a tendency to save energy. Over 30 minutes for example, you could walk at such a pace that you could be overtaken by a lame snail if such was your desire. You might only cover half a kilometre, or less! On the other hand if you set yourself 3–4 kilometres to walk, it doesn't matter how long you take because you're burning energy (and fat) irrespective of speed. And the more *inefficient* you are in moving your body through a medium, the more energy you'll burn (we'll come back to this later). In the very early stages, 3–4 km may be too much. You may just need once around the block, then twice, then three times, until you can cover at least 4 km each day, preferably seven days a week (but at least 6), and certainly trying not to miss two consecutive days.

The more inefficient *you are at moving your body through a medium, the more energy you'll burn.*

If walking is a problem, any other form of 'aerobic' exercise that uses large muscles of the body over an extended period will do. The ratio of swimming distance to walking is about 1:4 (that is, swim 1 km to equal 4 km walking); the ratio of cycling, around 5:1 (that is, ride 20 km to equal 4 km of walking). There are also other exercises that may be better for people with problems such as damaged knees, as is the case with many big men. Walking on a mini-trampoline, aquarobics, or even circuit training in a gym are alternatives. On a stationary bike you may have to set yourself to a time of say, 30–40 minutes, because the friction is not similar to that on the road and therefore distance covered is not always accurate. But when you have pedalled for that time once, you can then go for the distance covered next time. If you have an injury or illness such as arthritis, that makes most forms of movement difficult, your program will have to concentrate more on the energy input side of the waist control

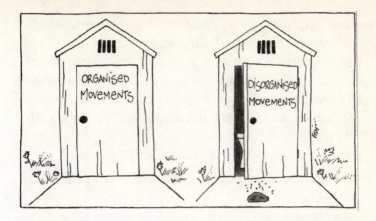

formula. Change the type and amount of food and drinks taken in to make sure of optimum benefits.

When to move

Organised or planned movement can happen at any time during the day or night. At least one man on the GutBuster Program enjoys his walk best at around one o'clock in the morning. There's little evidence that different times of the day have varying benefits on fat loss. Some people are 'morning people' and some don't start to wake up until the sun is well over the yard arm. That can also dictate when planned movement is most likely to be enjoyable—and remember, it MUST be enjoyable.

Hot or cold?

Winters can be cold, particularly in the mornings. And cold has the immediate effect of making you want to be warm. It's still a common belief that by rugging up

more—in 'sauna pants', track suits or rubber wet suits—
you'll sweat more and therefore lose more fat while
you exercise. Of course you may lose more *weight*.
But, as you know by now, *weight* is not necessarily
fat. Overheating during exercise can also be dangerous
because of the pressure it can put on someone with a
not overly well heart.

Why swimming is not a (good enough) waist of energy

Swimming is usually one of the first exercises on the
list of those recommended for fitness and fatness. But
while it may be good (if used properly) for fitness, there
are many reasons why it is less effective than other
forms of weight-bearing exercise for reducing fatness.
For example:

- Body weight is supported in the water, so less
  energy is required.
- Fat floats. So the fatter the individual, the less
  energy required to stay afloat and move in the
  water. This helps to explain why swimming is even
  less effective as a fat loss technique for women with
  their higher proportion of body fat.
- A lower centre of gravity and higher proportion of
  body fat helps females float better and therefore use
  less energy than men in the water.
- The rate of energy expenditure in the water
  depends on the efficiency of the swimmer. A very
  bad swimmer will burn more fat than a very good
  one. A good swimmer can also float along at a rate
  which has a minimal energy requirement.

- Maintenance of core body temperature during swimming is much easier than in land-based activities. Therefore energy is not required to keep the body cool or warm.

There are some benefits in swimming, particularly for the very overfat who have difficulty carrying out non-weight supportive activity.

Staying cool while you exercise may have some positive advantages. Professor Roy Shephard of Toronto University in Canada has found with soldiers in the Arctic that, even with a big increase in food intake, exercise in cold temperatures keeps fat down. The simple explanation for this is that the body uses up energy in the cold to maintain body heat. Walking on a cool winter morning with only light clothing, in contrast to overdressing, is likely to increase the rate of energy and fat burned to maintain body temperature. The moral here is to dress cool and let your body warm you up, not your clothes.

Other research has found that where the body is kept artificially cool during and after exercise, such as in swimming, there is less effort needed to return the body to core temperature. This effort also requires energy and could add to the fat-burning efforts of the exercise itself. This is not yet proven but it may provide

---

GB high energy tip

Dress cool for planned movement. More energy is required by the body to increase body heat during planned movement like walking in cool conditions wearing cool clothing.

further evidence against the efficiency of swimming as a fat-burning exercise and suggest that cooling down too quickly after organised movement, for example having a cool shower or a swim), may not be as effective for burning fat as allowing the body to cool itself down. Jumping under a cool shower immediately after exercising may also be dangerous because of the sudden changes in blood pressure.

Measuring your movement: phases 1 and 2--distance, then heart rate

In the first phase of any planned movement program for reducing body fat, the main concern should not be with intensity, as measured by heart rate, as in most fitness programs. Covering the distance is all that's needed. Walking or other exercise should be gentle and no more strained than a leisurely stroll—at least for the first 3–4 weeks. Concentrate on fitness once you have managed to reduce fatness. After the first month, though, you will notice your fitness level improving and you will have to increase the load to get the same benefits. This is where heart rate comes in, but with a different pulse rate to the complicated formula you may have seen up on gymnasium walls (that is 60–80 per cent of maximum heart rate (where MHR = 220 – age)). This formula is

---

GB high energy tip

Don't cool down too quickly. By making your body work to return to core temperature after exercise, more energy is burned up. A gradual cool down will also help prevent injury.

appropriate for *fitness*, but not for *fatness*. Fat is only burned in the presence of oxygen, as we'll see in the following chapter. The optimal amount of fat burn off occurs at around 120 heart beats per minute, depending on age (see Figure 9.1).

After your first month, try to walk the whole of your 4 km each day at an intensity that raises the heart rate to around 120 beats per minute (decreasing by about 10 beats for every decade over 40 years of age to 60).

> *Walking or other exercises should be gentle and no more strained than a leisurely stroll—at least for the first 3–4 weeks.*

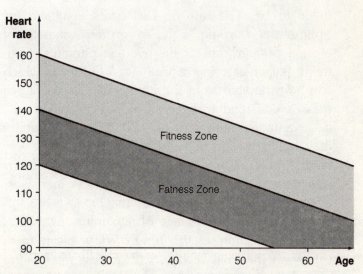

Figure 9.1 **Heart rates zones by age for increasing fitness and decreasing fatness**

Moving on: phase 3—Perceived ratings of exertion

After the first one or two months of walking, first aiming for a distance, then aiming for a particular heart rate, we now move to phase three: walking (or other-wise moving) to a feeling. Heart rate is useful. It can be used effectively on its own forever as your measure of effectiveness if you like. But it does have some disadvantages. For example:

1 *Heart rates change with age* The level of heart rate intensity for exercise efficiency is generally determined as a proportion of maximum heart rate (MHR). But maximum heart rate decreases with age (more so in some people than in others), so the older you become the less reliable this measure tends to be. The rate of 120 beats a minute for optimal fat burning is based on an estimate of around 50 per cent of the average person's maxi-mum oxygen-carrying capacity (or VO2 max.) which can be estimated from the heart rate. So you'll see that as you tend to become more 'chronologically disadvantaged', the rate of 120 beats per minute may not be giving you the best benefits.

2 *Heart rates change with fitness* Maximum heart rate depends on fitness level. As fitness increases, maximum pulse rate increases making it more dif-ficult to reach a percentage of maximum heart rate.

3 *Heart rates change with time of day* Heart rates vary with the time of day, with lowest rates being recorded around mid-afternoon. An exercise pulse of a certain percentage of maximum at this time of

the day might equate to a different level of exertion at another time of day.

4   *Heart rates change with medication*   Certain medications, particularly the beta blockers used for treating high blood pressure, tend to lower pulse rate and make it difficult to increase it with exertion.

What's the alternative to moving to heart rate? Swedish exercise physiologist Gunner Borg came up with one some time ago. He called it the 'perceived rate of exertion' or PRE scale. It began as a 20 point interval scale on which you rated your level of exertion from very, very easy, to very, very difficult. Borg has now modified this to a 10 point ratio scale as shown below.

To get optimal benefits from your planned movement sessions you might try walking at a rate of between 3 and 4, or between 'moderate' and 'somewhat strong'. Once you get used to the feeling at this

---

Perceived rate of exertion (PRE) scale

0	Nothing at all
0.5	Very, very weak
1	Very weak
2	Weak
3	Moderate
4	Somewhat strong
5	Strong
6	
7	Very strong
8	
9	
10	Very, very strong
	Maximal

level of exercise, there is no need to rely on pulse rate. Still keep to the distance, but you'll find that, as you get fitter, to get the best benefits you might have to add hills, soft sand, stairs, or even walk a longer distance to achieve that same level of exertion rated at 3–4.

Planned walking is really all the movement that is necessary for achieving and maintaining waist loss in men. Once you attain some degree of fitness and if you'd like to tone up, increase fitness or gain muscle by going to a gym, do so by all means. But if you're not an exercise lover, we can't stress enough that walking (with some stretching to maintain suppleness) is all that you need. Too many people fail on weight loss programs because they don't like the exercises they've been given to do and feel that they can't maintain them for a lifetime. According to the principles of the GutBuster Program, if you can't do what we're recommending for the rest of your life, don't bother.

Moving inefficiently—the best way to lose fat

It might sound a bit strange, but the best way to lose fat through movement is to make your movement *inefficient*. What do we mean by inefficient? We mean

---

GB high energy tip

Walk first for a set distance, then to a heart rate, then a feeling of exertion. As fitness develops, each of these measures of exertion guarantees optimal fat burning.

using more energy to do an activity because the body has not adapted to it.

A good example is the difference between walking and jogging. At around 7 km per hour, it's much more efficient (and therefore requires less energy) to jog at a slow pace than to walk briskly. Similarly, as one becomes adapted to carrying out a level of exercise at a certain degree of intensity, it becomes easier to do, and therefore requires less energy.

Body mass can also decrease with exercise over a certain period, and this can mean that less energy is burned, simply because it is easier to carry a smaller mass over a set distance. Let's take an example. A 100 kg man who is unfit will expend a lot of effort to walk one kilometre. Let's assume that he uses 100 Cals (4200 kJ) of energy. As he reduces his body mass to say, 80 kg, and increases his fitness level, the amount of energy required to cover the same distance could drop to 80–90 Cals (340–80 kJ).

Our man may now be burning a higher proportion of fat as his fuel source because he may now be working more aerobically, but the slight increase in fat burn off is not likely to be enough to compensate for the reduction in total energy expenditure. At this level, our sample man may have even 'plateaued out' because he's not burning enough energy to balance his food intake.

So, how do we get him back to burning more energy again? The answer is making his exercise effort once again more 'inefficient'. This can be done by increasing the intensity, frequency, duration, or even type of planned movement. Instead of walking quite

---

GB high energy tip

Vary your planned movement to maintain motivation.
Variation in activity between different aerobic exercises on
different days will ensure that staleness doesn't set in.

---

comfortably on the flat, the same man might now start
to add some hills. Instead of walking every day, he may
choose to swim, or ride a bike, or do something else
every other day. Instead of walking on a hard surface,
he may try walking in soft sand if a beach is close by.
Each of these factors will increase the difficulty of the
exercise and therefore the 'inefficiency' of the individual
in doing the exercise. If we increase *in*efficiency, we
increase the amount of energy used.

Acting your age

The notion of inefficiency also has implications for
ageing. Research carried out at Arizona State University
shows that walking at the same pace burns more energy
in older men (over 60 years) than in the young. Most
men choose to walk at the speed that is most econom-
ical for them, usually around 1.3 metres/second. At
this speed, older men burn around 15–20 per cent
more energy than younger men, possibly because of
the reduced efficiency of muscles with ageing. Pulse
rates also decrease with age and so the level of 120
beats per minute (bpm) for optimal fat burning becomes
more difficult to reach over the age of 40. The required
pulse level decreases by around 10 beats per decade
from age 40 to 60, so that a 50-year-old man would
only have to get the pulse to 110 bpm and a 60-year-

old to 100 bpm in order to get the same benefits that a younger man would get at 120 bpm.

What are the implications of all of this? As you get older, you don't have to walk as far, or as fast, to get the same fat loss benefits as when you were in your prime. In real terms, 2–2.5 km for the elderly would be the equivalent of 3 km for the young. Of course, the extra will always help if you can do it comfortably—and enjoy it! But it's worth knowing that some things don't have to stay hard all your life.

Putting all of this together we have the simple formula of planned activities and heart rate goals as shown in Table 9.2.

'Incidental' movement

We have considered the importance of 'incidental' movement previously, not only in burning extra energy but for its long-term effect of increasing metabolic rate. Little things, like not using the remote control on the

Table 9.2 A simple formula for planned movement

	Type of movement			
	Walking	*Cycling*	*Swimming*	*Other*
Frequency	daily	daily	daily	daily
Intensity				
1st month	slow	slow	slow	slow
2nd month	HR 120	HR 120	HR 120	HR 120
3rd month	PRE 5–6	PRE 5–6	PRE 5–6	PRE 5–6
Duration	3–4 kms	15–20 kms	3/4–1 km	30–40 mins

HR = Heart rate
PRE = Perceived Rate of Exertion

TV, mowing the lawn instead of paying someone else to do it, walking to the shops instead of driving etc., can all add to fat burning.

Now we want to add to this by suggesting that such movements (that were once thought of as being 'inconvenient' or a 'nuisance') need to be thought of as 'opportunities'. In other words, instead of thinking that having to walk to work during a transport strike is an 'inconvenience', see it as a way of burning up a little bit of extra fat. Instead of nagging the kids to get you something out of the fridge late at night when you're sitting watching TV, see it as interest on the fat you've saved yourself from storing during the day.

Everything that involves any form of movement should be seen as an *opportunity*, not an *inconvenience*. Unfortunately, we live in an energy-saving society which encourages us to even save our own energy. But, unlike power bills, this one builds up to be paid at a later date. Don't save body energy. Burn it.

Everything that involves any form of movement should be seen as an opportunity, not an inconvenience.

By *using* more energy, you'll also *have* more energy. Think of it this way: your energy supply is like a petrol tank, but a petrol tank that expands in size the more energy you take from it. If you're very unfit, your petrol tank may only have a capacity of 10 litres. Yet the limited amount of effort you need to get through the day uses up 9 of those litres, leaving you only 1 to spare for the things you'd LIKE to do, not just HAVE to do. As you use more energy, your tank will expand to say, 40 litres (these comparisons are similar to the increases that really happen). Now the extra moving that you're doing may use up 20 litres of that. That leaves another 20 to do the things that you want to, on top of the things you have to (e.g. see Figure 9.2)!

Now you may be able to see why a lean, fit athlete can do enough during the day to make your car feel tired, and still have plenty to spare to rage on into the night. A fat, unfit person on the other hand, may be dropping off to sleep during the day, and waking up constantly with sleep apnoea during the night.

Seeing movement in a different light

Movement is the key to fat loss, despite the lack of emphasis put on exercise by some more nutritionally-oriented 'experts'. Exercise should be seen as the key

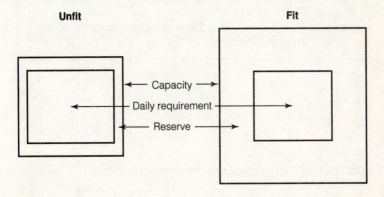

Figure 9.2

to major fat loss, not only because of the energy that's used up during exercise but also because of its effect on metabolism over the long term. Instead of seeing planned movement as a 'chore' it should be seen as *'time out'*; a time to relax, think, fantasise and escape the hassles of everyday life. Planned movement, seen in this light, not only has energy-burning effects but can also reduce stress which in turn can add to fat-burning benefits (see Chapter 15). In a similar vein, incidental movement needs to be regarded not only as an *opportunity* to burn up small amounts of energy but, more importantly, is also likely to increase metabolic rate over the longer term so that more energy is used up during the course of the day. Both of these approaches to movement require a significant shift in attitudes which are vital to long-term success in waist control.

GB high energy tip

Regard planned movement as a form of 'time out'. Instead of just exercise, movement should be seen as an opportunity to take time out, relax, think and remove oneself from the banalities of life.

---

10 The three energy systems: what's good for the goose, is not necessarily good for the gander

Some people are built for comfort, others for speed. And while this is true in a range of different areas, nowhere is it more true than in the way in which muscles work. There are indeed people who are built for long, endurance-type aerobic activity (the 'aerobes') and those more built for speed or power, like the Olympic weight-lifters (the 'anaerobes').

There are two aspects of this that are worth considering in terms of fat loss or energy gain. The first is the type of fuel that muscles may use best, and the second is the type of muscle that predominates in any individual. The implications are that some people may,

by an accident of birth, find it easier or harder to lose
fat and get fit than others. If so, it's worth knowing
this and the limitations that it places on you.

Fuel types and energy

Movement can only occur when muscles contract.
Because muscle is attached to bone, and most skeletal
muscle runs across at least one joint, contraction, or
shortening of a muscle, generally means one bone is
pulled closer to another via the intervening joint. Consider the biceps in the arm, for example. Although
strictly speaking this splits into two muscles (*bi* meaning
two), it has connections across the shoulder and across
the elbow joint. When the biceps contract, the forearm
is pulled towards the shoulder and the arm is bent.

Muscles are made up of thousands of long, thin
muscle cells, or 'myofibrils'. For a muscle to shorten,
these have to slide across each other, like a little
'tug-o'-war' team. For that to occur, energy must be
released in the muscle. This energy can come from
three sources. If a sudden, powerful movement is
required, there's not enough time for food energy to
travel through the bloodstream or out of the muscle to
power the action. There also won't be much oxygen
available to 'burn' the fuel, so the energy comes from
a source which is *anaerobic* (without air or oxygen),
and can only last for a short time. In this case, energy
comes from phosphates stored in the muscle cell itself.
The muscle has enough of these to perform an activity
that lasts for about 10 seconds, and they can recover
to their original level in about two minutes. Phosphates

power short, high-intensity forms of activity, such as leaping to your feet if a gun goes off behind you, or lifting a weight. This type of activity does not burn fat.

The second source of fuel is for action of a slightly longer duration. But this also has to power the muscles in the absence of oxygen and is therefore still anaerobic, because there is still not enough time for regular breathing to be involved. The fuel source is glucose from carbohydrate-rich foods which is stored in the muscle, liver and bloodstream. Under anaerobic conditions, glucose can power a muscle from around 45 seconds to 2 minutes. If there's still no oxygen at this point, the burning of glucose leads to a by-product called *lactic acid* which effectively stops the muscle from continuing to contract and therefore injuring itself. This energy system is called the *lactate system* and is involved in activities like 100–400 metre sprints, or short, sustained bursts of high-intensity activity. Again, very little fat is involved in the process.

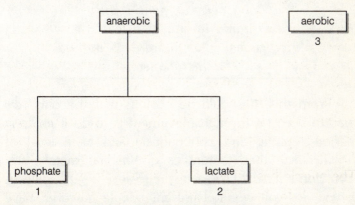

The three energy systems in movement

The first two sources are anaerobic, or operate without oxygen. The third energy source is the one from which we draw most of our energy and this is called the aerobic (with air) system. In this system, glucose and/or fat can be broken down to produce energy so that you are able to breath if oxygen is present. This type of energy normally powers our day-to-day movements and, under normal resting conditions, the ratio of carbohydrate to fat in the fuel mix is around 50:50. As we increase the *duration* of movement, the proportion of fat used increases so that the ratio may change to 80:20 (fat:carbohydrate). As *intensity* of exercise increases, the proportion of glucose increases to a ratio of carbohydrate:oxygen of 90:10, until, in a sprint, the activity ceases to be 'aerobic' and virtually all the fuel comes from carbohydrate.

The only real way to burn fat through movement is to do it for long periods, gently and continuously and at a level of 'inefficiency' that guarantees optimal fat metabolism.

From this, it should be obvious that the only real way to burn fat through movement is to do it for long periods, gently and continuously and at a level of 'inefficiency' that guarantees optimal fat metabolism. *You don't have to 'bust a gut to lose a gut'.* Indeed, if you do, you won't. Different people however, have different levels of fat-burning efficiency. Endurance athletes for example, pour more fat into the fuel mix right from the start, whereas someone who is very unfit and overfat would be working anaerobically at a very low level of intensity and therefore not burning much fat. Some people are also more suited to the longer type of endurance activity because of their genetic and physiological predispositions. In other words, some people are likely to be more effective 'fat burners'. The trick is to work out your optimal level and this can be determined from the PRE scale in Chapter 10.

Measuring fat use

If we burn different proportions of fat at different levels of exercise intensity, you may think it would be useful to have some device to measure this. It is possible. The metabolism of fats and carbohydrates uses up and gives off different levels of oxygen and carbon dioxide, so the ratio of oxygen breathed in to carbon dioxide breathed out can be used as an indication of whether the predominant fuel source is fat or carbohydrate. This is called the 'respiratory quotient' or RQ.

Until recently, measuring RQ has been complicated and required sophisticated equipment costing around $100 000, the type that's used for measuring fitness levels in expensive laboratories. Improvements in tech-

---

GB high energy tip

Remember you don't have to bust a gut to lose a gut. Anaerobic activity is not fat burning and is potentially dangerous for the fat or unfit.

nology have now allowed a small (5 kg) machine to be developed which can measure RQ through a simple tube you breath into. These machines cost around $10 000, but they may well become smaller and cheaper and find their way into the back pack of the future 'waist-watcher'. In the meantime, you'll just have to take our word for the fact that long, slow, continuous movement is more likely to lose a gut than vigorous, intense, infrequent exercise.

Muscle types

As well as muscles having different propensity for different types of energy use, the muscles themselves can be quite different, according to genetics and other factors. There are basically two types of muscle fibres: slow twitch and fast twitch.

Slow twitch These muscle fibres do not contract with a large degree of force, but are able to contract over a long period of time. This is the type of muscle that's generally associated with the longer, endurance type of exercise. Because these fibres are 'aerobic' they need oxygen, which is delivered in blood, and this generally gives them a darker and more reddish appearance than the fast twitch, anaerobic types of muscle tissue.

Fast twitch These fibres, on the other hand, contract powerfully, but are only able to do so for a limited period. Because they're predominantly anaerobic they run out of energy quickly. They are lighter in colour because they don't rely as much on oxygenated blood.

An example of the difference between fast and slow

twitch fibres in animals can be seen in the wings and legs of a chicken. The wings are designed to contract quickly and forcefully to get the bird into the air for a short period of time hence they have more fast twitch fibres and are generally white in appearance. The legs, on the other hand, have more slow twitch fibres that use oxygen for walking round for long periods and so are darker in colour.

Strangely enough, some people are built with a predominance of muscle fibres much like the chicken's wings, while in others the muscle fibres are more like the chicken's legs. Sprinters are generally fast twitch fibre types, whereas those who are better at longer distances have more slow twitch fibres. In most cases, it's difficult to change fast twitch into slow twitch fibre, or vice versa. Basically, you're stuck with the type of muscle fibres that you are born with. (One exception is a type of fibre called fast twitch IIA which can be conditioned for some types of endurance activity.)

We can see then that it is quite likely that the fat-burning capacity of different people will vary. Slow twitch muscle fibres contain more intramuscular fat and those who have a lot of this type of fibre can work aerobically over a long period of time. Since fat is burned in the presence of oxygen, it is likely that the

---

GB high energy tip

Understand your physical limitations and work within these. Muscle fibre types are relatively predetermined, setting limitations on performance in different types of activity.

aerobe is a more effective fat burner than the anaerobe. Recent research from the University of Sydney has shown that obese people do tend to have more fast twitch fibre. But whether this is a cause or effect of obesity is still not clear.

Fast twitch fibres also tend to grow more in response to resistance training exercises such as weight training and this helps to explain why some stocky males who are very effective in power sports can bulk up very quickly, whereas the leaner 'Jack Spratts' of the world could lift weights till the cows come home and still have muscles like chickens' insteps.

> *Some people are built for comfort and some for speed, and if this is the case, it's quite likely that the fat-burning capacity of different people will vary.*

This means that there are significant individual differences in the ways in which human beings perform physiologically, and also in the ways in which they gain and lose body fat. We've already mentioned genetics. Sex is another factor and energy systems and muscle fibre type are other factors which set limitations on what is possible.

Irrespective of energy systems and muscle type, fat is always metabolised through movement. You may think that you're doing plenty. But researchers have shown that individuals tend to overestimate the amount of exercise they are doing by around 40 per cent and underestimate the amount of food they are eating by around 30 per cent. Some people, especially fat people, underestimate how much they eat by even more. To see if you fit into this category, check your answers to the questions in the box below:

Testing your movement level

1 How often would you do any form of long, continuous movement (such as walking, jogging, swimming etc.)?

	Score
Rarely or never	1
1–2 days a week	2
3–4 days a week	3
More than 4 days a week	4

2 When you do this, how long would you usually do it for?

Rarely or never	1
Less than 15 minutes	2
15–30 minutes	3
More than 30 minutes	4

3 What level of intensity would you generally do this at?

Light
(e.g. slow walking, golf, gentle   1
cycling, bowls, doubles tennis)

Moderate
(e.g. brisk walking, cycling,   2
swimming, singles tennis)

Heavy
(e.g. jogging, squash, aerobics,   3
vigorous sports)

Scoring: Multiply your answer scores Q.1 × Q.2 × Q.3
1–8 Your level of movement is not sufficient for fat loss
9–18 Your level of movement can be increased
19+ Your level of movement is appropriate for fat loss

---

11 Turn on, trim down and drop it off

As our GutBusting Program tactics begin to have an effect, you might start to notice that there's something that appears to be alive under that mountain of slowly disappearing stomach flesh (apart from the dangly bits). You might remember it from your youth. It's called muscle. And now it's beginning to make its presence felt again, you might want to see and feel more of it—a touch of nostalgia from the old days. To do this we need to add some toning exercises to the fat burning we've been recommending so far. As we've said all along, movement (and exercise) for fitness is quite different from movement (and exercise) for fatness. In this chapter we'll look at the best and most efficient ways of toning muscle.

How not to 'bust a gut'

One of the most common exercise mistakes made by

men who set out to reduce fat is to begin weight training. In many cases they don't actually start, but *restart* something that they did in their youth—if it kept you trim, taut and terrific then, why not now? The problem is that weight training works muscle. There's very little call on fat as a source of energy when muscle is worked for short bursts very intensely, as in weight training. Fat, like petrol in a car, is used best when the whole body is moving.

Another typical mistake is to attempt 'spot reducing'. This means exercising a part of the body to try to reduce fat in that part. Sit-ups, for example, will work the abdominal muscles, but because they are not long-duration, low intensity effort, the energy for these muscles to contract is unlikely to come from any fat, let alone that particular fat lying over the abdominal muscles in the pot belly. A fat man who only does sit-ups is therefore likely to wind up with a *tight* fat belly instead of a *loose* fat belly, but little else!

Fat is mobilised best through whole body movement. Once the belly starts to disappear though, there may then be reason to begin to tone the muscles underneath. Sit-ups and other types of toning exercises can be built into a program after 3–6 months of fat-burning activity.

GB high energy tip

Forget about sit-ups unless you can feel muscle on your stomach—not just fat. Sit-ups may tighten muscle underneath fat, but what's the point if the fat is not reduced so that you can see it.

Toning and calisthenics

Compared with walking, most men find calisthenic or
weight training type exercises boring. If this is the case,
that's fine. Don't do them. Remember, any change has
to be one that can be done for the rest of your life.
For the man who wants a little more for his money,
these exercises can help restore a little muscle tone and
strength and may also add to the metabolic effects of
aerobic exercise by increasing the proportion of the
energy-burning muscle mass of the body.

There is also a compromise. For anyone concerned
with fatness rather than fitness, a lot of time spent on
calisthenic type exercises could be a waste of time. So
we recommend a limited exercise program to help tone
up the muscles that are probably in most disrepair,
usually the abdominals and muscles in the lower back.
The following simple toning routine can be *combined
with* (but not substituted for) any movement program.
These exercises should be carried out after walking or
other warm-up movements.

Exercises for working the abdominals and lower back

Crunches

The best known exercise for the abdominals is the
crunch or sit-up. It is typically done wrongly. Because
the abdominal muscles flex the upper body towards the
hips, any movement that locks the legs to the floor will
not work the abdomen but the hip flexor muscles that
run from the upper thigh to the lower back. The first

principle is to never lock the feet by holding them under a bed or table. The hips should be flexed by bending the knees and keeping the feet as flat on the floor as possible. Other tips for the sit-up (or curl-up) are as follows:

- Tuck the feet under the buttocks.
- Dig the heels into the ground. This flexes the hamstrings which are antagonist to the hip flexors and therefore relaxes these more.
- Tilt the pelvis so there is no arch between the lower back and the floor.
- Place the hands lightly on the ears or forehead.
- Slowly roll the upper body (do not jerk the head) only as far as it will go with feet remaining flat on the floor.

Do 5–10 sit-ups at a time initially, then add to this number as the effort becomes less.

Sit-up and twist

Once you have mastered the sit-up, an addition can help extend the effort to the muscles at the side of the waist (commonly called 'love handles'). This time, as you raise the upper body off the floor:

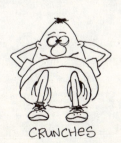

CRUNCHES

- Twist the upper body so that the right elbow touches the left thigh (it may not actually touch, but that's the general direction).
- Slowly return to the start position, then curl up twisting the left elbow towards the right knee.

Add twisting to the sit-up routine as it becomes easier to do.

Reverse curls

Sit-ups work the upper abdominals. To ensure a full abdominal-strengthening work-out using the lower abdominals as well, the trunk should be flexed from the lower body with reverse curls or leg raises. *Do not attempt this exercise if you have a bad back*.

Lie on your back on the floor with your hands in the small of the back for support. Now, slowly roll the legs (knees bent) towards the chest, raising the buttocks off the floor as knees near the chest. Hold for 1–2 seconds, then slowly return. Do not straighten the legs at any time as this will put extra pressure on the back. Do 3 to 5 of these, then up to 20 as the stomach increases in strength.

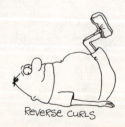

REVERSE CURLS

Back extensions

All exercises should be balanced, and so when working one muscle group exercises for opposing muscle groups are necessary to ensure no imbalance. The opposing muscles to the abdominals are in the lower back and it is these which often cause problems in men with large bellies and weak stomach muscles. Strengthening of the lower back must be done with caution and should *not* be done without instruction from a qualified person if you have a back problem. Consult your doctor or back specialist *first*.

To work the lower back muscles, lie face down on the floor. Slowly raise the right arm and left leg off the ground and hold for 4–5 seconds, making sure the limbs are not hyper-extended and taken too far. Slowly lower, then repeat with the left arm and right leg. Use opposing arms and legs to guarantee minimal pressure on the lower back. Carry out 3 to 5 of these exercises initially, then build up as your back becomes stronger.

Circuit training

Circuit training is one of the oldest forms of calisthenic exercises around and it resurfaced in recent times in the form of the Canadian 10BX and 5BX programs. It involves carrying out a number of exercises in a sequence over an extended period so that fat is being burned through 'aerobic' exercise and the specific muscles being worked are both toned and strengthened. Circuit training is useful for keeping to your movement program when the weather is too diabolical for outside walking, or if you're stuck in a confined space such as a hotel room somewhere on business and would like a nice compact little exercise program. The sample circuit below can be used successfully for fat burning and toning in these circumstances provided the following conditions are adhered to:

- Continue moving between exercise stations.
- Carry out several repetitions of each exercise before moving to the next.
- Once a round of exercises has been completed once, do it again (2–3 times) to get the extra benefit.
- Try to ensure that any circuit keeps you moving for at least 20 minutes.
- Combine exercises so that the same group of muscles is not being used in consecutive exercises.

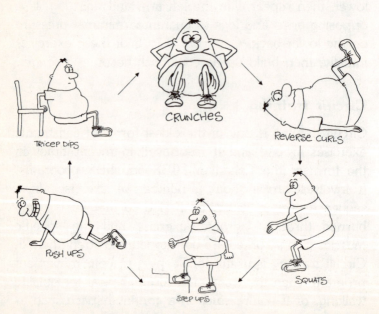

Stretching the point

One of the disadvantages of continuous aerobic exercise such as walking is that muscles are contracted within a limited range of movement. Consider the hamstrings at the back of the thighs, for example. These muscles (there are three of them) are stretched when the leg is extended. But they are hardly stretched to their limit during walking, because the leg is rarely extended more than about 30° past the vertical. On the other hand, these muscles are continuously contracted when the knee is bent during striding. If the hamstrings aren't stretched after walking they are likely to shorten and tighten and ultimately cause problems with flexibility at a later time. Stretching of the main muscles used in any activity such as walking should therefore be part of any exercise program to maintain flexibility and prevent injury. There are three main stretches that are important for walking and these should be done for 10 to 20 seconds each, before, but even more importantly after, a planned movement such as walking.

Hamstring stretch

This can be carried out either sitting on the floor or standing up. Straighten one leg and slowly bend the upper body to reach as far down the straight leg as

---

GB high energy tip

Stretch yourself. Always stretch before and after walking to stop muscles and tendons shortening and causing potential tightness or injury.

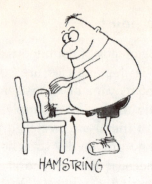

HAMSTRING

possible. Never go past a point of pain. Hold for 10 to 20 seconds, then repeat with the other leg.

Calf stretch

The calf muscles (gastrocnemius) are used to contract the foot during walking and should therefore be kept flexible through to the Achilles tendon which joins the calf muscle to the heel. The calf is stretched by straightening the leg and holding this action, as in the common 'tree pushing over' action seen by runners warming up before a race. Under the calf, a second muscle called the soleus also plays a role in flexion of the lower limb and this can be stretched by a slight variation on a calf stretch just by bending the knee.

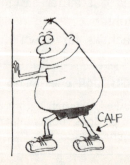

CALF

Anterior lower limb stretch

Having stretched the back of the leg (calf and hamstrings), the front of the lower leg should also be stretched to prevent 'shin splints', pain in the front of the leg which often occurs when heavy men initially take up a walking program. The peroneal muscles which run up the front of the lower leg can be stretched through the action shown in the diagram below. Hold for 10 to 20 seconds and then repeat with the other leg. Make sure that the toes are tucked under so that the stretch is felt in the front of the leg.

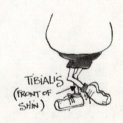

IV
Learning how to behave —again!

12 Pattern interruption and behaviour modification

Apart from genetic, racial and gender factors, being fat and unfit basically comes from improper eating and/or too little movement. So why, if we know this, and we know the dangers of being fat, do people let it happen? Hedonism is an obvious reason. It feels good to stuff your face with lots of creamy, sugary and fatty foods. It also seems bad, or appears so for some, to spend any energy trying to balance this food input with exercise output in movement, when there are all sorts of machines around to do things for us.

Another less obvious reason is that much of what we do, we do out of habit, without thinking about it. Habits are nature's way of helping us to do all the things we have to do in a day without having to waste time thinking about them. They help us do basic chores—eating, dressing, sleeping, driving—on 'automatic pilot', so that we can occupy valuable mental space with more enlivening topics.

Habits are nature's way of helping us to do all the things we have to do without having to waste time thinking about them.

Russian psychologist, Ivan Pavlov, first demonstrated simple or 'classical' conditioning with the famous Pavlov's dog experiment. When Pavlov presented meat to a dog, it salivated in anticipation of eating. When he then paired the presentation of the meat with a bell, it wasn't long before the bell alone was enough to lead to salivation. The meat was called an 'unconditioned stimulus' (US) and the bell a 'conditioned stimulus' (CS). By continual pairings, the CS became all that was needed to lead to a conditioned response (CR). The dog had learned to salivate at the sound of a bell. This then formed a *pattern* of behaviour which happened automatically as long as the CR led to a reward which reinforced the behaviour.

Classical conditioning is only one way in which behavioural patterns or habits, are formed. But it is perhaps the best illustration of how this can happen. It shows how easy it can be to literally expand before your own eyes—without your brain ever realising what is happening! Fattening habits, such as always finishing a meal, eating at set times of the day whether you're hungry or not, collapsing after a meal to watch TV, eating chips or peanuts with beer, are all done on cue to a conditioned stimulus, just as Pavlov's dog salivated on cue to the sound of a bell. Although Rover's salivation has a life-saving function, for humans some of these conditioned responses tend to become much less functional than they might be under different survival conditions.

Habits can be behavioural or cognitive. Behavioural habits are those that occur automatically and involve little cognitive (thinking) involvement. These are the type of negative behavioural patterns that are mostly associated with male obesity and lack of fitness. Cognitive habits, on the other hand, are learned patterns of wrong thinking, including conditioned thoughts of depression, failure, worthlessness, frustration and unrealistic ideals. These are more characteristic of females with weight control problems who have suffered a lifetime of pressure to conform to social and media stereotypes. Dealing with cognitive habits involves detailed psychological techniques which will not be covered here. Changing behavioural habits means interrupting patterns of behaviour through modifying the stimulus–response relation. This is considered in more detail in this chapter.

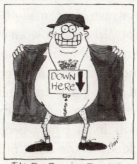

THE POT BELLIED FLASHER

Pattern interruption and behaviour modification

Men and women are different when it comes to behaviour associated with health. Look at diets, for instance. How many women regularly go on diets? How many men, on the other hand, do you think feel guilty, worthless or totally inadequate if they don't stay on the weekly women's magazine diets that would hardly provide enough energy for a marsupial mouse? The answer is likely to be very few.

It's true that women are the victims of social pressures to conform to an unrealistic body stereotype. There is also little doubt that this results in extremes of eating disorders as mentioned earlier. (Interestingly, the male equivalent is more likely to be body building or body bulking.) There is also little doubt that these pressures make women *think* differently from men about body shape, fat loss and fat gain, and the behaviours associated with these. What we're alluding to is that fat gain and loss for women is much more of a thinking, or cognitive process. It involves destructive thought patterns that work against any simple change in energy input or output that would normally be associated with changes in body fat. Whereas a woman on a diet might know that there are roughly 500 Calories (2100 kJ) in a slice of cake and think that she really must not eat it, then eats it and feels guilty and inadequate for doing so, a man will generally just eat the cake—because the occasion calls for it! In fact he's become conditioned, often without thinking, to the habit of say, sitting down to a cup of tea with a piece of cake, drinking alcohol with a bag of crisps at hand, eating snacks while watching TV ads and many similar conditioned responses.

'. . . *women* think *differently from men about body shape.*'

As we said previously in Chapter 3, successful female fat loss programs call for changes in thinking patterns about eating, exercise and self—a difficult and often detailed task. Men, on the other hand, are much simpler beings. Their programs generally require an understanding of simple pattern formation and learning how to break the stimulus–response bonds that have formed over many years.

Stimulus–response (S–R) bonds

Behaviour modification is designed to change learned behaviour patterns so that future, more healthful behaviour patterns become part of day-to-day life and are therefore easier to carry out. Pattern interruption is the term used for the process by which these S–R relationships are broken. The process is as follows:

1 Recognise the pattern that has formed. This is done, as was pointed out in the *GutBuster Waist Loss Guide*, by 'stalking' habits as a hunter stalks his prey.
2 By stalking the habit (pattern) it should then be possible to determine the conditions under which it occurs (for example, being in a bar, going out to dinner, after some drinks).

3   Once the pattern is recognised, it then needs to be
    interrupted by either changing the conditions or
    purposefully modifying the response. (For example,
    either keep out of the bar or don't have a drink in
    the bar, don't go out to dinner, or be conscious of
    choosing something different at dinner.)

Because a habit is an automatic response to a given
set of cues, in theory, all that has to be done to change
or learn something different (once you become aware
of the habit) is to repeat another chosen (healthy)
pattern over and over again until *it* becomes automatic.
Eventually you substitute the newly acquired habit for
the less desirable one. In practice, of course, this is not
as simple as it sounds because attitudes, belief systems
and social pressures interfere with the relearning process. In general, however, the process in men does not
seem to be as complicated in this respect as it is for
women and so simple pattern interruption can be quite
effective.

Pattern interruptus

The key to behaviour modification is *pattern interruption*. This must be done on a regular basis so that any
negative pattern of behaviour is broken. In the case of

GB high energy tip

Stalk your habits until you are aware of them. Becoming
consciously aware of when, what, how and why you are
doing something is the first stage of breaking the pattern
of response that leads to fatness and ill-health.

Pavlov's dog, for example, the association between the bell and salivation was broken by simply presenting the bell several times without the food. In other words, the conditioned stimulus, because it is eventually unrewarded, no longer remains a conditioned stimulus. This leads to what psychologists call 'extinction' of a behaviour. In an example of food being eaten every day with morning tea, the equivalent process of change would be:

1   dissociating the food from the tea;
2   not having morning tea at all;
3   replacing the food with something else (such as a low-fat food) until such time as there is no longer an association between morning tea and eating.

This form of action involves removing the stimulus.

This process of pattern formation and interruption can be summarised as in the box below:

Stimulus–response relationships

US or unconditioned stimulus (meat) $\longrightarrow$ UR or unconditioned response (salivation)

CS or conditioned stimulus (bell) $\longrightarrow$ CR or conditioned response (salivation)

A similar form of pattern development in humans may be:

Food presentation $\longrightarrow$ Eating
Morning tea time $\longrightarrow$

A second way of interrupting patterns is to change the response (R) associated with the unconditioned stimulus. In the case of the morning tea example, this would mean doing something else other than eating when morning tea comes around, for example, going for a walk, continuing to work, playing with worry beads etc., until such time as the old behaviour pattern has been interrupted to the extent that a new and more constructive pattern has formed.

There are four main processes that can aid in pattern interruption: self-monitoring, stimulus control, response management and reinforcement

Self-monitoring

Research shows that self-monitoring of eating and exercise-related behaviour increases the chances of fat loss. We know that most people underestimate the amount of food they eat and overestimate the amount of exercise they do. The only way to become aware of this is to self-monitor by writing down every food eaten and every exercise undertaken. In some women's programs the individual also adds how they 'felt' at the time of eating (e.g. depressed or happy), but this does not seem to be as important for men. Simply writing down *everything* that is eaten or drunk and *every* extra bit of exercise (as in the GutBuster exercise and diet diary) is enough. Another way of self-monitoring is to use measurement devices like a pedometer for measuring distance walked. One brand of pedometer now on the market even measures energy 'in' (food and drink) and equates this with energy 'out' from movement to automatically give an energy balance estimate at the end of the day. In the future, as we have noted, there

> **GB high energy tip**
>
> *Watch yourself.* Monitoring behaviour helps you to understand that behaviour in a more effective way. Write down what you eat and what you do daily to make sure that these are fully understood.

may also be small machines for measuring fat metabolism through RQ measures.

Pulse rates, waist size and other measurements can also be regularly monitored.

> **Self-monitoring**
>
> • THINK before eating (even place a THINK sign on the fridge).
> • Keep an eating diary and identify triggers for eating.
> • Keep an exercise diary.
> • Measure waist size, resting pulse and distance walked regularly.
> • Use exercise-recording devices such as a pedometer if desired.
> • Examine patterns in your eating.
> • Chart your progress in an obvious place (e.g. on the fridge).

Stimulus control

As was seen from the discussion earlier, it's a conditioned stimulus (CS) which elicits an automatic, or conditioned response (CR). If the stimulus is absent, the response is much less likely to occur. Stimulus control therefore, can occur through:

1   *Limiting exposure* to the stimulus (e.g. if socialising

causes you to eat more fatty foods, the level of socialising might need to be reduced).

2 *Manipulating* the stimulus (e.g. socialise at home where fatty foods are not available).

Stimulus control

In social situations
- Don't drink alcohol while eating—have it before or after meals.
- Have a glass of water, cup of tea etc. instead of a second helping.
- Have a drink after a meal that doesn't go with dessert, e.g. beer instead of ice cream.
- Go to restaurants where there are more low-fat choices (e.g. Japanese, Thai).
- Park away from a restaurant and walk to and from it.
- Focus on your behaviour rather than your weight.
- Plan high-risk situations in advance.

Home
- Alter the antecedents (or stimulants) to eating.
- Store foods out of sight.
- Eat meals off a smaller plate.
- Do not clean your plate—try to always leave something.
- Cover your plate with a napkin when finished.
- At a buffet, allow yourself only one trip to the food and/or use only a small plate.
- Distinguish hunger from cravings and ignore cravings.

Drinking
- Don't start drinking until a set time (e.g. 6 p.m.).
- Have at least one or two alcohol-free days each week.
- Don't drink while eating.
- Keep worry beads/keys in your pocket to occupy your hands.
- Keep peanuts or chips out of arms' reach.

---

3   *Interrupting* the stimulus–response connection (e.g. play with worry beads or chew gum when socialising so that you don't over-eat).

Some examples of stimulus control under various situations are given on the previous page.

Response management

This involves manipulating the response which occurs to a conditioned stimulus. The first stage is to develop an awareness that the actual response is associated with the stimulus. The second stage is to provide alternatives to that response (for example, if socialising causes drinking, substitute low-calorie drinks, or do something else with your hands). A third possibility is to force yourself not to carry out that response on repeated occasions, until it becomes 'extinguished' and is no longer automatically connected to the stimulus.

Response management

- 'Stalk' your habits.
- Interrupt your eating behaviour chains.
- Learn relaxation.
- Put your knife and fork down between bites.
- Combine water/mineral water chasers with alcohol.
- Have an alternative exercise planned for cold/wet days.
- Organise a friend or partner to exercise with you so that you can't renege.
- Plan walking/exercise in advance (for example, arrange to meet a friend or neighbour for an early morning walk).
- Ban the words 'must', 'should' or 'ought to' from your vocabulary about relapses.

Reinforcement

Reinforcement, or 'reward', is a way of ensuring that a more desirable response will become associated with a stimulus. Rewarding oneself for a good week (e.g. by buying some new clothes or allowing yourself a drink on Friday night) will reinforce positive behaviour and reduce the chances of negative behaviour occurring. Some examples are given below.

Men's weekly habits: it's downhill from Monday morning

Behaviour patterns are not only developed in small units: they sometimes form weekly and even yearly ways of responding. A recent survey of eating patterns in Australia, for example, showed some interesting short and long-term patterns in eating over the working week. The survey found that dietary patterns close to that regarded as healthy (such as eating breakfast and eating low-fat and high-fibre foods with limited alcohol consumption) are most common in men on Monday

---

Reinforcement

- Set short-term goals (behaviour as well as achievement).
- Set incentives for yourself for reaching these.
- Involve your partner.
- Tell your partner how to help.
- Set incentives with your partner (sex/holidays etc.).
- Reward yourself for *doing* things, not just *achieving* things.

mornings. After that, it's a progressive downhill run to Sunday night.

As the week progresses, men:

- are less likely to eat breakfast;
- eat more take-aways;
- drink more alcohol and soft drink;
- eat more sweets or desserts;
- eat more cakes and biscuits.

Weekends are the time for greater consumption of:

- bacon and eggs;
- alcohol—wine and beer;
- pizzas, hamburgers and other take-aways.

Shown graphically, changes in healthy behaviour patterns from Monday to Sunday could be represented as shown in Figure 12.1.

You could probably also substitute the months of the year for Monday to Sunday. The beginning of the year is always time for a new start. But as the year progresses, and particularly towards Christmas, healthy behaviour patterns rapidly decline culminating, for many, in the gross over-indulgences of Christmas dinner.

Most weight control programs designed for women aim for perfection by levelling off the squiggly lines shown in Figure 12.1—attempting to make everyone perfect (and boring) for the week, the year and a lifetime! Naturally they rarely work, as hedonism usually triumphs over masochism. Any program for men, then, should take into account varying dietary restraint during

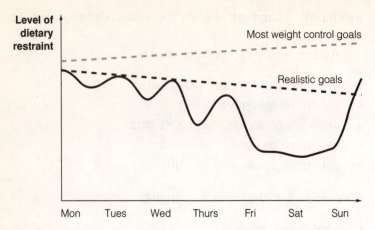

Figure 12.1 Level of daily and weekly restraint in men

the week and the fact that weekends seem to be associated with a release of inhibitions.

Weekends appear to serve a psychological, perhaps even stress-relieving, function (see Part 6). If goals are set too high, they're bound to fail. Programs should be built into the weekly cycle, making modifications where it is easier to do so (that is during the early part of the week) rather than attempting to counteract established lifestyle patterns. The realistic approach to high energy health—while not becoming a boring old fart—is to

---

GB high energy tip

Extend the week till Friday night. It's now well known that men's best intentions are blown away on weekends (as at the end of the year). So trade off by restraining yourself earlier in the week and then enjoying the week-end.

trade off the excesses of the weekend by response modifications such as:

- Extending the week to Friday night.
- Having at least two alcohol-free days early in the week.
- Not drinking alcohol before 6 p.m.
- Trading off Sunday lunch (if this is desired) with extra walking or reduced fat intake.
- Trading off weekend evening indulgences with extra walking.
- Limiting fatty breakfasts (e.g. bacon and eggs) to Sunday morning only (if at all).

Denial, distraction and distortion—the delusion of the 3 Ds in managing health behaviour

In his book *Act Thin, Stay Thin*, Dr Richard Stuart explains that we often confuse what we would like to do with what we actually do. Stuart outlines three sources of delusion—denial, distraction and distortion—which help to explain why some people sometimes over-eat and under-exercise without necessarily knowing that they do so.

GB high energy tip

Try not to drink alcohol before 6 p.m. One of the main health risks of alcohol is its promotion of unhealthy eating habits. Delaying the start of drinking delays the possibility of this.

Denial

This is a useful defence mechanism because it helps us maintain a positive image of ourselves. We can't live happily without it. But when denial becomes excessive, it can lead to self-defeating behaviour. If someone denies their eating excesses, for example, there is little chance of overcoming these. With eating, the main form of denial is denying that you ate too much. With exercise, it's denying that you *don't* do enough regular activity. The usual response is 'I'm on my feet all day'. Overcoming this requires honest understanding as well as some objective measurements (such as pedometer scores, food diaries, etc.) that cannot be denied.

Distraction

This occurs when other things are happening. It's easier to eat too much, for example, while having a drink or talking with friends. It's easier to automatically eat while distracted by watching TV. Research has shown that overweight people are more vulnerable to distractions than normal weight people. When the distractions are aroused emotions, the effect is even greater. Researchers have shown that when obese and non-obese people are left in a room with open access to food, and with a clock in view which is sped up so that 50 minutes represents an hour, fat people eat when they think it's *time* to eat (e.g. 1.00 p.m., although it may really only be 12.00 p.m.). Non-fat people eat *when they feel hungry*. They're not distracted by the time.

Distortion

This refers to the way in which overweight people judge their eating behaviour. Studies recently reported in the UK using radio-isotopic methods to measure *actual* food intake and exercise output and equating this with *reported* food intake and exercise output have shown that overweight people underestimate food intake by around 30 per cent and overestimate exercise by around 40 per cent. This is not thought to be deliberate (because even normal weight people do it). It's an unrecognised *distortion* of the facts. They're just unaware of the amount they actually eat.

You cannot make sound plans for effective behaviour change when you start from where you think you'd like to be instead of where you really are.

Distortion with eating refers to a misperception of what is eaten. 'I only had a small piece' or 'I only drink occasionally'. With exercise, distortion refers to a mis-perception of what exercise involves: 'I play tennis twice a week' (therefore I do a lot of exercise).

Self-monitoring can help you overcome the triple threats of denial, distraction and distortion because, according to Dr Richard Stuart '. . . you cannot make sound plans for effective behaviour change when you start from where you think you'd like to be instead of where you really are'.

GB high energy tip

Don't plan to change without changing the plan. Being aware of the causes of fatness and ill-health is only the first step. Plan a pattern interruption program around these to do something about it.

Summary

In theory, pattern interruption as summed up here seems simple. In practice, however, it involves large hunks of motivation. And motivation, as we all know, is dynamic, with highs and lows, plateaus and dips. It's vital therefore to understand these processes in order to guarantee the long-term success of your waist loss program.

V

Getting the get up and go to get up and keep going

13 Getting the get up and go

Motivation, says the Macquarie dictionary, is '. . . *that which prompts a person to act in a certain way*'. But motivation is dynamic, not static. Everyone has had the feeling of leaping out of bed one day and feeling like turning over a whole new branch, then falling out the next day barely able to pick up the rotting leaves. Everyone—even the world's most dedicated athletes— suffers ups and downs, peaks and gullies, in their desire to strive for and achieve certain goals. Unfortunately for some, the peaks are mole hills and the gullies feel like ravines at times, making long-term changes in body fatness difficult, if not impossible.

Motivation for long-term health, then, has to be not just '. . . *that which prompts a person to act . . .*' but that which also *continues to* prompt a person to act in a certain way over an extended period of time. By its very dynamism, the things that motivate are likely to change over time. Anyone who has travelled the road from total sloth to high-level wellness is aware that there are landmarks along the way. Some are lucky enough to have experienced these, but few have been able to enunciate them—at least in Western societies— possibly because of the difficulty that scientists have in associating physiological states with psychological feeling.

The landmarks will include psychological stages of well-being, plateaus in improvements and psychological 'downers'—these are inevitable stepping stones in the body's striving for greater physiological and psychological well-being. Part of the battle is in understanding these psychological signposts and in using them to further increase motivation and push the process closer to final goal achievement. Another part of the battle in overcoming barriers is through an awareness of what they are and how to break through them, by physically 'shocking the system'—creating new goals and new targets at higher levels of achievement.

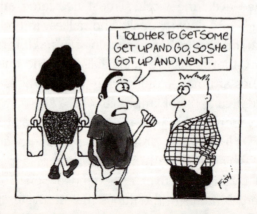

All the world's a stage

Have you ever wondered how long-distance runners ever get the motivation to keep it up? Why fanatical tennis players will risk anything to bash a little furry ball over a net? Why dedicated surfers will go through hell and cold water to find the perfect wave?

The answer is not just enjoyment, but what psychologist Mihalyi Csikzentmihalyi (we'll call him Dr C) calls *flow*. This happens when one experiences even simple activities as acutely psychologically rewarding— similar to a form of meditation or a 'high' (the term 'runner's high', for example). The characteristics of this flow are:

- loss of the sense of time;
- merging of action and awareness;
- acute well-being;
- analgesia to mild pain;
- disappearance of ego awareness;
- detachment;
- a feeling of freedom.

Of course these things don't happen overnight. When they do, you'll probably never look back. The only motivation that is necessary then is 'intrinsic'—it comes from within and is an attempt to recapture the sheer pleasure of the peak experience. It keeps runners running, tennis players tennising (!) and surfers surfing.

According to Dr C, *flow* occurs within a channel that is dependent on two main parameters—one related to the task difficulty, the other to the competence of the performer. This is summarised in Figure 13.1.

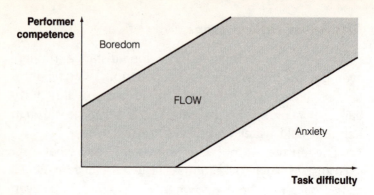

Figure 13.1

In the situation where the difficulty of the task exceeds the competence of the person carrying out that task, a situation of anxiety arises. Let's say, in our case of regular movement, that you're unfit but try to do something vigorous—say running—that requires a high level of fitness. Anxiety, distress and extreme fatigue are likely to be the result. The implications? Get fitter or go slower.

At the other extreme, a highly competent performer faced with an easy task will get bored quite quickly. Imagine walking at a snail's pace when you're a marathon runner. The response may be beneficial healthwise, but it's hardly likely to turn you on psycho- logically.

In the shaded area shown in Figure 13.1, competence and task difficulty are so matched that a *flow* pattern occurs such that the performer and the environment interact. This happens when you become so involved in an activity that you enjoy and feel comfortable doing, that things around you can become blurred and you become merged with the activity. Your walking (or other form of movement) and even your whole lifestyle now takes on a psychological component as well as being physiological—it becomes intrinsically rewarding to the extent that you enjoy doing it for its own sake. At this stage you'll begin to look forward to the health changes you've made and feel disappointed if, for any reason, you have to go without the activity.

Stages of motivation

It is the ultimate goal of any lifestyle-based program to get to the stage where changes are enjoyed so much that they can't be done without. But there are other stages on the road to this point. Three can be identified, together with their own practical implications for pushing you towards the point of no return—where you no longer need to be motivated because it has become a way of life.

Stage 1: Discomfort

For the overfat (and usually very unfit), the first thing that's felt on exerting effort (such as in walking) is discomfort. You've probably been through this by now and so it needs little elaboration. In physiological terms, it means that aerobic fitness is not well developed and energy is mainly metabolised anaerobically. This causes

---

GB high energy tip

Design your program to 'go with the flow'. Any severe changes in lifestyle will cause anxiety that, in turn, will mean that they can't be maintained for a lifetime. Work at a level that causes neither anxiety nor boredom.

a shortage of wind and thus discomfort. The duration of this stage will depend on individual levels of fitness, previous exercise experience, physique and type of exercise. It can take from two to ten weeks of regular gradual exercise to get through this stage.

In relation to changes in food intake, a similar process can occur. Cutting back on fat in the diet can be a rather drastic step. You'll feel cranky, dissatisfied and irritable. However, you should be aware that it won't always feel like this. And if you increase fibre, at least you won't feel hungry. Most lifestyle changes—decreasing salt intake, increasing fibre, decreasing sugar and fats and increasing movement—take at least 2-3 weeks before you begin to enjoy them. As anyone who has stopped adding sugar to their tea or coffee will tell you though, once this initial stage of discomfort has gone, you may find it hard to imagine going back. In most cases its the changes you make which seem more 'natural', not the behaviours you've changed from.

Within this stage, we can also identify some sub-stages as landmarks along the way.

Maladaption This is where the body tends to react adversely to the unusual demands being put on it, even if these are introduced gradually. In relation to extra movement, such as walking, this may result in stiffness

---

GB high energy tip

Persist with any changes made for at least 2-3 weeks. Research shows that any lifestyle change requires time but, with persistence, reverting to previous habits then becomes difficult.

and soreness initially, but if the movement is carried out gradually and accompanied by stretching, the degree of stiffness and soreness should be minimal. The initial period of maladaption relating to dietary changes will be characterised by a craving for those foods (particularly fats) to which the body has grown accustomed. The process is maladaptive because it doesn't happen simply. It's also likely to be uncomfortable for a time; at least until the body begins to adapt.

Gradual adaptation This is where there is no longer stiffness and soreness from movement or craving and hunger for foods, but it's still not enjoyable and hardly seems worth the effort. The individual at this point will need TLC (tender loving care) and plenty of 'extrinsic' motivation to help him get through this stage without becoming disillusioned. It is at this point in the GutBuster Program, for example, where a heavy reliance is put on group support and regular (i.e. weekly) group meetings to maintain motivation. Those having completed the introductory stage of the program, or the first GutBuster book, will generally have progressed through this stage.

Stage 2: physical comfort

After a certain amount of graduated movement and improved healthy eating anyone can begin to benefit. Most men will move to this stage quickly when they start walking (i.e within 1–2 weeks). This is probably as a result of an increased aerobic capacity which makes the effort feel worthwhile. The feelings most often spoken about are a warm, tingling muscular sensation AFTER exercise, improved sleep and metabolic function, loss of fat and a sense of physical satisfaction. In terms of dietary changes, the loss of high-energy dense and fatty foods from the diet has now become more bearable and you may even be beginning to feel the physical benefits such as a reduction in gastric 'reflux' reactions, fewer feelings of 'bloatedness' and less post-prandial (after meal) fatigue, particularly in the middle of the day.

Again we can identify two sub-stages.

Exertion At this point exercise and changes in the diet are still demanding and sometimes difficult to stick to, but it begins to feels good AFTER having made the effort. You might also find that you begin to feel bad when you fall down and fail to carry your commitment out—if you miss your daily walk, or over-eat on a high-calorie meal. There's still little 'intrinsic' reward, though, and most of the good feelings which come from achievement are physical and not psychological.

Relief At this point, movement is accompanied more by a sense of muscular relief and relaxation. Your daily walk will begin to not only feel good, but also to be something that you look forward to, and miss if you don't have. Although the rewards may still not be 'intrinsic' or occur *during* the exertion, there's enough benefit from the day-to-day feeling of improved physical well-being *afterwards* for you to want to continue. Dietary changes also begin to feel good physically. There may be a growing sense of satisfaction with a lower level of 'fullness' or satiation than you remember from your less inhibited days and you may feel a sense of relief in now being in control of your food intake rather than being controlled by it.

For many, this might be the final stage of achievement with fat loss and improved fitness. And it could be enough. By now there's a feeling of 'intrinsic' or internal reward from your actions which is likely to keep you going along the same track. For others there could be further joys in store as the physical satisfaction turns to more psychological satisfaction with continuing gains.

Stage 3: psychological rewards and emotional 'highs'

Although not everyone gets there, it's generally accepted that there can be a third stage of lifestyle improvement where this becomes 'addictive' with feelings of 'highs' or 'peak experiences'. This is generally most characteristic of aerobic exercise and is one of the reasons for using movement instead of diet as a means of fat loss. Still, where exercise like this is combined with a healthy—low-fat, high-fibre—diet, the 'highs' can tend to be even more rewarding and may be enough to encourage you to seek more. It's the reason why joggers continue to run long distances in the face of what many people would think is a painful experience. There have been suggestions that the highs at this stage are related to a release of 'endorphins'—the body's natural opiates—in the brain. Again, there are sub-stages to look for.

Psychological satisfaction At this stage exercise is enjoyed for its own sake. It feels good WHILE YOU ARE

DOING IT. You may even find yourself looking forward to exercise and enjoying it more.

Consciousness expansion At this point, the activity becomes its own reward and little outside encouragement is necessary. You'll know the feeling and you'll always want to get back there. Runners talk of a 'flow' experience and creativity seems to be increased DURING the activity. There is also a loss of self and a type of meditative effect.

Not everyone will get to this stage, particularly those maintaining only a low level of health related activity. However, it's worth striving for because, at this point, the psychological rewards become so satisfying that little else is needed for maintenance of this type of program for a lifetime. This is the stage called *flow* by

Table 13.1 *Stages of motivation*

Stage	Sub-stage	Feelings
1 Discomfort	Maladaption	Discomfort, out of breath, pain, desire to stop.
	Gradual adaptation	Decreased muscle soreness, reduced exertion.
2 Physical comfort	Exertion	Physical demand but sense of achievement.
	Relief	Muscular relief and relaxation, feeling of physical satisfaction.
3 Psychological	Psychological satisfaction	Well-being and feeling 'at peace' with the world; relaxation.
	Consciousness expansion	Euphoria; consciousness change; feeling of 'high'; loss of sense of time.

GB high energy tip

Be proud of your achievements—not yourself. A castle
built on self esteem can come crumbling down at the first
stumble. Be proud (or disappointed) of your achievements,
not yourself.

Dr C and the goal of any high energy wellness program
even though it may not be necessary for someone to
reach this stage in order to gain the long-term benefits
of a high energy lifestyle.

Getting onto the stage

Now that you're aware of the various stages and pitfalls
that you're likely to go through in your quest for
reacquaintance with some long forgotten body parts,
you're likely to be interested in some techniques for
getting through those stages. Of course, the hardest
part of any program is the first part, that is the
discomfort stage. Once through this, however, not only
will your physical performance improve, but so will your
psychological attitude. By our definition, it's the discomfort stage where 'extrinsic' motivation is most necessary, because doing what you're doing doesn't yet
feel good in itself. Some examples of extrinsic motivation that may be useful include the following.

Be aware of plateaus, 'downers' and stages

To help you through the hardest stages you need to
know that things are going to get better. It won't always
be like this. Improvements may come within a day, a
week or a month. But they will come. They may also

be transitory, with some good days and bad days. However, provided that you're on the right track, the former will soon begin to outweigh the latter.

Set short-term goals

A loss of 1 per cent of waist per week is a good start. After the first 1–2 months this might start to slow down as it becomes harder and harder to shock the body into giving up its spare food supply. A 1 per cent reduction each fortnight might become a more realistic expectation, although many men achieve more than this.

It is also important to set broader process (as opposed to outcome) goals to maintain motivation. These can include such things as reduced weekly fat intake and/or increased fibre intake (as measured with your fat and fibre counter), establishment of 1–2 alcohol-free days per week, reducing food intake on social occasions, etc. Resting pulse and even blood pressure changes are other short-term measures that can be used for motivation.

Add variety

Although walking and reduced dietary fat are the keys to the GutBuster Program, the introduction of variety—the unfamiliar—can help to increase performance by increasing energy expenditure and changing energy input. Eating a wide variety of foods, including some you may never have tried before (provided that they are low fat), is likely to not only help you physically but also to add a little spice (literally) to your life.

Plan ahead

Instead of only thinking about what to do for exercise and food intake on the day that it happens, plan this in detail the night before. That way you are less likely to renege. You may be surprised, but some of the busiest people in the world build their daily health activities into their diary and refuse to change these unless under the most exceptional circumstances. Remember, if you fail to plan, you plan to fail.

Record

Self-monitoring is one of the best forms of motivation, as well as useful for planning behaviour change, as we have seen in Chapter 12. Keep records of a range of factors that indicate improvements, not only in outcome, but in process. For example, resting pulse, exercise pulse, waist size, distances walked, calorie input etc. Monitoring equipment such as pedometers and computers are now available to assist this process.

Reward

A life of waist loss doesn't mean a life of drudgery. We know, and expect, that men are likely to forego their good intentions as the week progresses, so this can be used to your advantage. For a week that has been 'extended to Friday night' it's quite OK to reward yourself with a good night out, a social event or a good old piss-up. Other rewards might be clothes, a weekend away, a holiday on the money you've saved, or something else you may have wanted for some time (no need to tell anybody else).

Use the 'mate' system

Peer pressure is a great form of motivation. Line up with a mate or your partner to walk at a certain time each day, talk about and check your eating patterns, or do other recreational activities together that involve movement for fat loss. If your mate is female, however, it's worth making sure that both you and she are aware that her fat losses may not be as quick or as successful as yours for all those reasons explained in Chapter 3.

Use fantasy and imagination

One of the main benefits of exercise is its value as a stress reducer or a form of 'time out' from daily anxieties. Regular walking, jogging, cycling or swimming can be useful forms of mental relaxation where fantasy, imagination and creativity come to the fore. Many runners, for example, use this time to create; businesspeople use it to work—and even dictate into a hand-held micro-recorder—because this is the time at which they are at their most productive. Use your mind to think, create and expand by letting it run free.

14 Plateaus, downers and 'shocking the system'

There's a saying *'you can lead a horse to water . . .'*. Unfortunately, it's not always true. The horse may not want to be led—thirsty or not—just like a rotund man may not be motivated to shed fat. Even if he is, there'll almost certainly come a time when the urge will wane. So getting it up and keeping it up becomes a multi-skill in the middle years.

The fact that you've picked up this book (and presumably the one before it) implies that getting the urge up is not likely to be the main problem. If you're like most men in the GutBuster Program, you're probably driven by the feeling of discomfort that carrying a rucksack full of T-bone steak trimmings around your middle can bring. You may also have hidden in the back of your mind the health consequences of that and the desire to live past a time you may not see if you keep on the same downhill toboggan ride.

Whatever your motive, you're now here. The challenge is to keep you here—in sickness and in health, for richer or for poorer, till death do part you and your belly. For this to happen, you'll need to understand not only the stages along the way, but the fact that fat loss may 'plateau'; the psychological 'downers' that inevitably occur from time to time; and the urges that say 'stuff it' every now and then when temptation presents itself.

Fat loss plateaus

Anyone who has tried to lose fat knows the frustration of hitting a 'plateau'—a point at which no further fat loss seems to be occurring even though diet and exercise are still being controlled.

What is a plateau? And what can be done about it?

Plateaus are entirely natural in any loss of body mass. They're a result of the body's adaptation to changing energy demands which may last for a period of days, weeks, or even months. A plateau can occur as a result of the body becoming more 'efficient' in managing restrictions that have been put upon it. For example, for anybody exercising and using the same routine for

---

GB high energy tip

Focus on your behaviour, not your weight. Behaviour changes will ultimately lead to health improvements, but focusing only on the outcome can make you take your eye off the ball.

a long period, efficiency in carrying this out is improved. Hence the energy required (that is calories used up) decreases. Similarly with food intake. Metabolism, like everything else, gets better with practice. So the energy required for the digestion of a particular food is likely to decrease as that food becomes more familiar.

Plateaus arise from the body's adaptation to changing energy demands as a result of the body becoming more 'efficient' in managing restrictions that have been put upon it.

The first thing in dealing with plateaus is to accept the fact that this is a normal and natural process. Provided that there's no increase in fat mass, the plateau can be countered by attacking the causes, that is, improved efficiency. Because plateauing results from the body 'becoming used to' the changes you've instituted, breaking through a plateau requires 'shocking the system' to make it 'unused' to new changes and once more 'inefficient' thereby requiring more energy to carry out the activity).

GB high energy tip

'Shock' the system to get through plateaus. Plateaus are a natural process of the body adapting to change. Breaking through these requires 'shocking the system' to make it unused to new levels of activity.

Shocking the system

In terms of exercise load 'shocking the system' means making exercise less efficient by changing:

- Intensity—increase the speed at which the exercise is carried out.
- Distance—exercise over longer distances.
- Frequency—exercise more regularly (e.g. by adding 'incidental' exercise).
- Type—vary walking with cycling, swimming, aerobics, etc.

With food intake as the other side of the energy equation, the system can be shocked and plateaus can be countered by:

- Decreasing calorie intake—but only where this is still high.
- Increasing calorie intake—by refeeding where calorie intake is excessively low (i.e. under 1000 Cals/day, 4200 kJ/day) and has been for long periods.
- Decreasing fat intake further—to reduce appetite for fat as well as calorie intake.
- Changing food type—eating foods that the body is unfamiliar with.

Plateaus are the scourge of the waist-watcher. However, they needn't be if their cause is acknowledged and appropriate steps taken.

Psychological 'downers'

Along with the inevitable plateaus in fat loss come the

inevitable periods of 'bugger it, what the heck', that is, lapses in motivation. These might coincide with a couple of big nights out, some inclement weather, or nothing obvious.

Again, it's important to realise that psychological downers are perfectly natural. Motivation is a dynamic, not a static variable. There will be times (for example, when you begin the program) when motivation is extremely high. There will also be times when it's not so high, and times when it's lower than an ant's instep. If you are aware of these times, you can take the necessary steps to recover. If you're not aware, and one day of inaction or indulgence stretches into another and another and another, recovery will become harder and harder and harder—being directly related to the length of time of relapse.

By all means, then, have a day off if you feel the need; be a little more cautious about having two consecutive days off, and try not to ever have three. Some of the techniques for motivating yourself through and past these downers are pointed out at the end of this chapter. The big concern is where a motivational 'downer' meets a plateau, as shown in Figure 14.1.

This is where warning bells should ring if you don't want to waste all the effort that you've put in so far. To begin with, make the three Ps clear in your own mind: that this state is neither permanent, personal or pervasive.

By *permanence* we mean that all plateaus have a finite time-span. They may be a week, a month, or 6 months. But generally they end with a movement off the plateau, either up or down. It's important to make

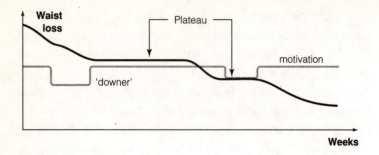

Figure 14.1

sure that it's down (provided the plateau is not your goal waist size). In the meantime, and during any plateauing phase, just be content that you are not increasing in size.

Not being *personal* means that this doesn't happpen just to you. Plateaus in fat loss (and even gain) are physiological facts characteristic of most animal species. Psychological downers, or at least changes in the levels of motivation, are also quite normal and should be expected.

Not being *pervasive* means that plateaus and downers should be seen for just what they are—plateaus and downers. They should not pervade your whole program to the extent that you think that nothing is working, that it's bigger than you can handle and that your failure will interfere with all other aspects of your life.

GB high energy tip

Regard plateaus and downers as inevitable. These are common to everybody and are the body's way of naturally adapting. Just be sure that you don't lose ground.

Come to accept plateaus and downers as a necessary dynamic of any fat loss program. If you do this, you can then see their solution—'shocking the system'—as an integral part of your shift to a goal waist size.

VI
Being overstressed for the occasion

15 Why stress and body fat?

Ask any group of men what aspect of health they would like to know most about and the answer will invariably be 'stress'. But the GutBuster Program is about fat bellies. So what has that got to do with stress?

Strangely enough, quite a lot. In a roundabout sort of way, not only can stress cause men to *store* extra fat in the fat cells around their middles but, once it's there, stressful situations can actually *release* the fat back into the bloodstream—and this is potentially dangerous. Your doctor may not believe this. But this is how it happens.

Why stress causes fat

Under cases of severe life-threatening stress, most animals (including humans) stop eating and soil their jocks—literally! Fortunately, this type of stress usually doesn't last for long. The type of stress that we encounter daily, however, does. It's frustrating, annoying and interferes with your life, but it's usually not life threatening.

Not only can being fat and unfit make you stressed, but being stressed can make you fat and unfit.

Under these circumstances a lot of humans—particularly fat ones—don't stop eating. They eat more. In fact, we know that those who are regarded as 'restrained eaters' (e.g. those who restrict their food intake because of consciousness of being too fat) tend to be the worst offenders under stress. The first thing they do is eat more. Restrained eating, and all other concerns about food intake go by the wayside. For this reason, stress can increase fatness and decrease fitness. Long-term, 'chronic' stress can do the following:

- *Encourage nervous over-eating* In some people stress can decrease the appetite, but in others it makes them pig out to the max! It's not just something to do with those nervous hands: food provides a kind of comfort—it feels good—when all about you might feel bad.
- *Increase alcohol consumption* Alcohol is a great way to 'blot out' the effects of stress. After a few grogs you can fantasise about what you'd like to do to solve your problems. The trouble is, it doesn't last. Alcohol is a short-term solution to stress, but it can lead to long-term fat belly problems.
- *Immobilise the body* Feeling like not wanting to

move is a symptom of severe or chronic stress. Not moving means not burning up calories. Not burning up calories means getting fat. Animals that are put in continued stressful situations from which they can't escape, actually give up and become totally immobilised. This syndrome is called 'learned helplessness' by psychologists. Similar things can happen to humans.

- *Decrease feelings of 'self-control'* The loss of control over one's life, as we'll see in the next chapter, is one of the main symptoms (and causes) of stress. If this flows through to other aspects of life, loss of control over waist loss and health practices will also occur.

- *Increase mobilisation of fatty acids* One of the (apparent) benefits of stress in fat loss is that it mobilises fats from fat stores to be used as energy. However, if there's no accompanying movement or exercise to use up this fat, it will remain in the bloodstream and can clog arteries and cause heart problems. This is one of the main health ill-effects of stress.

- *Decrease 'self-esteem'* For many individuals, an increase in stress leads to a reduction in self-esteem which then flows through to all other aspects of life—including fat control.

Why fat causes stress

In men, the result of all of these fat building factors is often a fat belly. This is because it is the belly where men store that excess energy—in a readily accessible form so that it can be squirted into the bloodstream to provide an extra source of energy to the muscles when needed. And it's a very good source of extra energy. While the blood sugars, the most immediate and accessible form of energy for muscle tissue, provide only enough energy to last for around 10 hours, the reserve stores in body fat will keep you alive for between 20 to 30 days! (It also helps you float if you happen to fall overboard at sea.)

Fat is brought into the energy cycle as a result of need. If you've eaten less energy than you're using up—in other words, if the body is in negative energy balance—more fat will be released, just as savings are used up when you run out of cash. One of the key factors that stimulates this process is the action of catecholamines (hormones from the adrenal glands), such as adrenalin and cortisol.

Catecholamines also happen to be the key hormones associated with the stress response. Everyone knows about 'adrenalin rush'. But you may not know that it's this that is vital in any stress situation to get your heart pumping, to tense your muscles, increase your breathing rate and increase sweating in readiness for cooling of the body—in short, to prepare you for the 'flight' or 'fight' that's needed to escape from a 'stressor'.

The difference between stress and straight exercise, however, is that these days stress is usually *not* accompanied by physical activity. There's no 'flight' or 'fight' to burn up all the energy from the fat that is being poured into the bloodstream. And this is the problem. The fat hangs around in the bloodstream where it can clog up the arteries just as mud might clog up a hose. Meanwhile the heart is pumping fifty to the dozen, putting all sorts of pressure on what is, in many cases, an unfit muscle. And, just like an unfit muscle, it might eventually give up the ghost.

It should be clear by now that not only can stress cause fat, but fat (particularly the spare tyre variety) can also cause a fair bit of stress. This is particularly so with relation to the heart and the heart is one organ that does not cope very well under these circumstances. So understanding and relieving stress *is* an issue that is of particular relevance to getting rid of a pot belly and regaining high level energy. The big questions are 'what is stress', and 'what can you do about it'?

All stressed up and nowhere to go

Stress is the non-specific response a body makes to a stressor. Why *non-specific*? Because, unlike a specific reaction to, say, touching something hot, which is a quick withdrawal of the hand, the stress response is a general bodily reaction to all outside demands.

Stress is a very individual thing. A stressor for one person—let's say arguing a point with someone—can be a delight for others. The job of an ambulance officer, from the outside, would seem to be a pretty stressful one, but most ambulance officers seem to not only cope, they even thrive on it. Yet, when they go home, they may find that the stress of a crying baby is more than they can handle. For someone else, it's the other way round.

Professor Hans Selye, the Canadian endocrinologist

acknowledged as one of the world's leading experts on stress, says that stress itself is not a problem. 'Stress', says Selye, 'depends not on what happens to an individual but upon the way he reacts'. We all seek an optimal level of stress in our day-to-day lives. If there's none, boredom sets in. If there's too much it becomes crippling.

Stress, then, is an outcome not a cause. It is dependent on two things: first a 'stressor', or stimulus, and second a 'stressee', or respondent. But stress is not a simple outcome of the matching of a *stressor* with a *stressee* as is clear from the description by Professor Selye above. Stress is a function of the *perceived* (not necessarily actual) demands made by the stressor, and the *perceived* (not necessarily actual) self-capability of the stressee to deal with the stressor. This is then appraised in the mind of the stressee and if there is a negative imbalance, that is, if the demands are greater than the capability of the stressee, stress results. In other words, stress results from the way in which a person *thinks* about, perceives or reacts to a stressor. This is shown in diagrammatic form in Figure 15.1.

Types of stressors for an individual can be either acute or chronic. Some examples of each of these are shown in Table 15.1.

Table 15.1 suggests that there is a big psychological component to stress—and that is true. But there is also a physiological component associated with those psychological feelings and both of these have to be managed in dealing with stress.

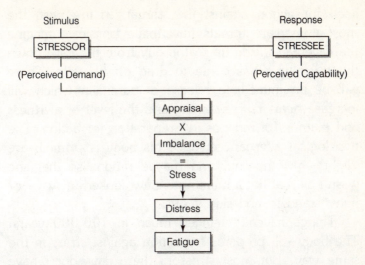

Figure 15.1 Causes and outcomes of stress

Stressed to kill

The first thing that happens in response to a stressor is a feeling of threat—either physical, mental or emotional. Once this happens the body prepares to defend

Table 15.1   Levels of stress and stressors

		Stressors	
Type of stressor	Severity	Physical examples	Psychological examples
Acute	Mild	Caught on a busy road	Being abused by driver
	Severe	Carried out to sea in a rip	Witnessing a disturbing event
Chronic	Mild	Drought for a farmer	Work
	Severe	War	Relationship problems

itself for action against that threat. In the past, the most immediate threats have been physical: imagine the caveman facing up to the guy from the cave down the track who has come to drag off his wife. There will be an immediate release of adrenalin which will increase heart rate, sweating and the level of alertness and tautness of muscles in preparation for action. The two logical alternatives, once his body is primed, are 'flight'—give her up, and maybe rationalise that she wasn't all that hot a mammoth stew cooker anyway—or fight: stand to and slug it out.

Things haven't changed much in 100 000 years. The body still prepares for action against stress in the same way. But most stressors these days don't have such clear cut alternatives for solutions: it is just not kosher to flatten the boss when he's pressuring you—or to run away. Yet that's what your body is ready to do. It's all stressed up, with nowhere to go. Muscles become tense and tight and then fail to relax. This tightness is increased with every undealt-with stressor.

The main muscles which are affected are those known as 'preparatory' muscles which prepare the body for either flight or fight. The trapezius (from shoulders to neck) raise the arms and shoulders in preparation for physical attack or defence; the abdominals tense to protect against a blow to the solar plexus; the gluteals

---

GB high energy tip

Plan for high-risk situations in advance. Forewarned is usually forearmed. Plan how you'll handle the high-risk party or business lunch in advance.

prepare for possible evasive action, e.g. departing the scene quickly; and the lower back muscles are tensed for postural stability in a crisis.

You can test the tension in these muscles by digging the tips of your fingers or thumbs into them at the points shown in Figure 15.2. If the muscle is tense and tight, there will be some pain even with minimal pressure. Soreness suggests a need for stress reduction or relaxation initiatives—escapes—such as those discussed later in this and the next chapter.

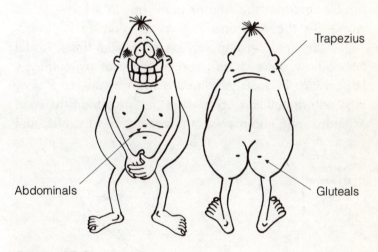

Figure 15.2

Time out as a 'de-stressor'

Often these physiological reactions to a stressor occur almost imperceptibly. Researchers in Sweden, for example, have shown a gradual build-up in stress-related hormones on an almost linear basis in employees who work extended time with no leave. The build-up happens in the way shown in the top line of Figure 15.3. When time off is taken (for example, weekends), these hormones decline to a lower level and then start to build up when work re-starts.

You can see this yourself by the aggro that builds up in business towards the end of the week. Friday is a bummer of a day because by that time everybody has built up a head of steam in their work and wants what they want done—today! By Monday, of course, the pressure's off. So much so that some people have trouble getting the momentum up to even get to work—it's the syndrome known as 'Mondayitis'.

A similar thing happens on an annual basis. You'll notice how, towards the end of the year, everything's happening. People have moved from a walk to a slow jog and are building up to a sprint. Drivers on the road are impatient; shoppers in the streets are frustrated and

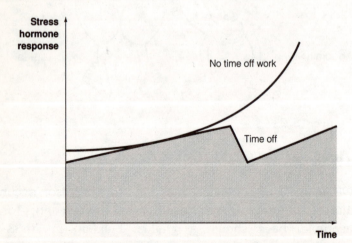

Figure 15.3 The build-up of stress-related hormones with and without regular time off work

pushy; workers in the workplace are irritable. At this time, there's a fair bit of pressure-cooker releasing going on by way of the artificial de-stressors provided by numerous Christmas parties. But these only cause a few stumbles on the race to the line. Then, on Christmas Day, it's all over. Compare the Christmas Eve tension with that of Boxing Day and right through January. In most Christian countries you could drop a bomb and nobody would care very much. It seems that if somebody's God didn't give us weekends and Christmas as periods for de-stressing, we'd have to invent them!

And it's not just humans that behave in this way. Psychologists working with rats several years ago, found that they could be encouraged to accept an alcoholic drink. But the time they liked it most was when they were put into a stressful situation (e.g. impending electric shock) and made to work to avoid this for a certain period, then given some time off. After they learned when to expect their stress period to end (the equivalent to a human weekend), they tended to hit the grog more. It's called the 'Friday night syndrome' and it helps to explain why there are more fights, murders, alcohol abuse and car accidents on Friday nights.

Stress, then, is a natural human reaction. In proper perspective it has survival value for the species. Too little can make life dull and uninteresting and decrease performance. But too much can be depressing and debilitating and also decrease performance. As we've seen, it can also make you fat—or at least stop you from becoming thin.

16 Why politicians have long lives—or does it just seem that way?

The one word that stands out in any discussion of stress is 'control'. A stressor is not stressful if you have control over it or, perhaps more importantly, if you *think* that you have control over it. It's only when *perceived* control either decreases or is absent that stress ever becomes a health issue.

Imagine, for example, flying a hang glider—probably a stressful experience for many people. For the experienced flyer, on the other hand it's a breeze, because he has control of the situation. Now what happens if he hits an updraft of wind, or is suddenly flipped over: if the pilot *feels* as though he's lost control, the situation can become quite stressful, even for the best of budding birdmen.

Take a more chronic situation—pressure at work.

While you are *coping* with orders and pressures and demands, there's probably not much of a problem. In fact, many people regard a bit of pressure as exciting. But what happens when the orders bank up, you can't fulfil them, people are demanding their problem be looked at, and you're the one who's getting blamed. It's difficult under these circumstances to have control over other people's actions and it may be these that add to the stress.

There are big individual differences in levels of control. The ambulance officer discussed in the last chapter is in control in the helping situation, but may not be in interpersonal relationships. Politicians who you might think would be extremely stressed given the weight of all our worries on their shoulders, seem to thrive on the pressure—while they're in control! They even seem to live longer—look at Mao Tse Tung, Genghis Khan, Winston Churchill. Not the healthiest of lifestyles, but ones which assumed a large degree of control. The loss of control, for example when politicians are thrown out of power, can be more stressful than the stress of lots of pressure with lots of control.

ACT on stress

The main point about 'flight and fight' as reactions to a stressor is that they enable us to regain control. Another strategy for regaining control has been described by the late Dr George Sheehan (the American 'running' guru) as 'negotiation'—the 'flight' come 'fight' of modern man. Sheehan claimed that you can tell by looking at a man's body shape whether he is built for

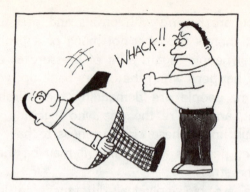

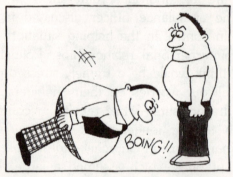

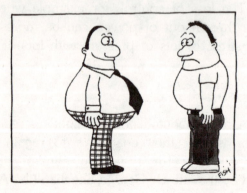

WHY POLITICIANS HAVE A POT BELLY.

flight, fight or negotiation. All, however, imply regaining control. And to the extent that control can be learned, the following tips can be useful:

- Build resistance to stress by regular sleep, exercise and good nutrition.
- Withdraw physically from a stressful situation for a while.
- Have regular breaks—weekends and holidays.
- Recognise your own optimal stress level and aim to keep below it.
- Learn a technique of mental 'escape' (see below) for when you can't escape physically.
- Practise saying 'no'—nicely.
- Believe that you can do something about stress.

Re-establishing control obviously requires more than these glib 'do this' statements that you might read in any anti-stress manual. It means understanding the complexities of both stressors and stressees and the most appropriate ways of changing these to correct the imbalance between *perceived demand* and *perceived capability*, as discussed in the previous chapter. A simple three-stage approach to this is outlined in Figure 16.1 and Table 16.1.

The first stage is Analysis. This requires an understanding of the distinction between the stimulus (stressor) and response (stressee). A stressor can be either actual (e.g. war, drought, famine) or imaginary (e.g. an anticipated outcome). The appropriateness of the response will depend on the type and intensity of the stressor—real or imaginary. A stressee can be affected by a stressor depending on his level of

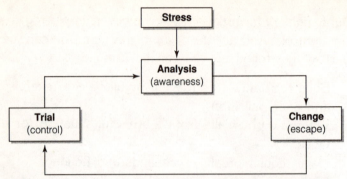

Figure 16.1 The ACT system for dealing with stress

'hardiness' to stress (see below) and the way he perceives the stressor (cognition). The effects of this can be shown in many different ways—psychological (e.g. anxiety, fatigue), physiological (e.g. sweating, elevated blood pressure), or pathological (e.g. allergy, disease).

Table 16.1   Approaches to dealing with stress—the ACT model

		Source of stress	
		Stressor	Stressee
Analyse		Type	Type
		Source	Effects
		Intensity	Response
Change		Reduce	Flight
		Remove	Fight
		Replace	Freeze
		Re-structure	
Trial		Measure	Measure
		Monitor	Monitor
			Master

Often the effects of stress build up so slowly that they are unnoticeable until they are made conscious.

The second stage of dealing with stress requires Change. This is necessary to restore control, or at least the *perception* of control. Changing the stressor can involve removing, replacing or restructuring it through either engineering or social engineering processes. The stress of excessive noise in the work environment, for example, can be relieved by engineering processes that reduce or eliminate it; family stressors can be changed by processes like family therapy, which involve social engineering. Changing the stressee involves two main approaches to dealing with stress—flight or fight—and applying each of these appropriately to the situation. A third alternative, 'freeze' or resignation, is the result of defeat and submission.

The notion of 'flight' is best encompassed in the term 'escape', which can be accomplished in either a mental or physical sense. 'Fight', on the other hand, doesn't necessarily mean physically attacking a stressor (although this can be a de-stressing tactic in some situations). It can apply as much to the fight that goes on internally with thought processes that are destructive and stressful. As Shakespeare once said in *Hamlet*: '. . . *things are neither good nor bad, but thinking makes it so*'. Fighting stress then can involve restructuring thought processes as much as escaping from these. The principle here is ' . . . *if you can't change the situation, change the way you think about it*'.

In this chapter we deal with 'flight', both mental and physical, and how this can be effective in changing stressful situations. In Chapter 17 we discuss 'fight', or dealing with internal conflict and the benefits of this in more intransigent stress situations, where it becomes necessary to change the way the situation is viewed.

Escape: the key to regaining control

Looked at in logical terms, the most effective approaches for re-establishing control, whether *real* or *perceived*, involve some form of 'escape'—either mental or physical. Physical escapes are those things that you can do to (a) either get out of the situation or (b) relieve the tension in 'preparatory' muscles by relaxing them in some physical way, such as through

Table 16.2   'Escapes' (flight or fight) from stress

	'Flight'		'Fight'	
	Physical	*Mental*	*Physical*	*Mental*
Maladaptive				
	Alcohol	Mind control	Violence	Blame
	Drugs	Cultism	Displacement	
		Denial		
		Negativism		
Adaptive				
	Exercise	Meditation	Negotiation	Cognitive restruc.
	Sport	Muscle relaxation	Confrontation	R.E.T.
	Warm baths	Prayer	Challenge	Assertiveness
	Holidays	Concentration	Preparation	Change
	Mini breaks	Counting to 10	Engineering	Psychotherapy
	Hobbies	Art	Social	Time control
	Games	Mind games	engineering	Finance control
	Yoga	Music	Nutrition	Positive self talk
	Tai Chi	Creativity	Direct action	Rehearsal
	Breathing	Reading	Meeting	Thought stopping
	Sex	Trance		

exercise or just bashing the bejesus out of something. Mental escapes involve processes such as progressive muscular relaxation, meditation, concentration or even prayer—things that enable one to take a 'mental holiday' from a stressor. Some of the easiest, but artificial 'escapes', such as drugs or alcohol, have the disadvantage under this schema of not *restoring*, but *removing* control. These are not effective long-term remedies. Some examples of different forms of escape are shown in Table 16.2.

GB high energy tip

Learn your best method(s) of 'escape'. The most effective forms of stress management involve some form of 'escape'—mental or physical. Knowing your best technique will help you solve your upcoming stresses.

Escape is a technique used by us all at some time. Yet, as with individual reactions to stressors, there are differences in people's suitability for different forms of escape. Some people are best suited to physical escapes such as sport or exercise, whereas others are more suited to mental escapes such as relaxation, meditation, or movies. Some can do both. The test shown in the box on the next page is one way of determining which is the best type for you.

If you score highest on 'physical', you're more likely to succeed using the physical 'escapes' as a means of coping with stress. If you score highest on 'mental' you may be more suited to using a mental approach. Progressive muscular training is one of the most com-

Stress test

Rate the degree to which you generally or typically experience each of the following symptoms when you feel anxious or stressed.

		Not at all				Very much
A	I have difficulty concentrating because of uncontrollable thoughts	1	2	3	4	5
B	My heart beats faster	1	2	3	4	5
C	I worry too much over something that doesn't matter	1	2	3	4	5
D	I imagine terrifying scenes	1	2	3	4	5
E	I feel jittery in my body	1	2	3	4	5
F	I get diarrhoea	1	2	3	4	5
G	I can't keep anxiety-provoking pictures out of my mind	1	2	3	4	5
H	I feel tense in the stomach	1	2	3	4	5
I	Unimportant things bother me	1	2	3	4	5
J	I feel like I am losing out because I can't make up my mind quickly	1	2	3	4	5
K	I pace nervously	1	2	3	4	5
L	I become immobilised	1	2	3	4	5
M	I perspire	1	2	3	4	5
N	I can't keep anxiety-provoking thoughts out of my mind	1	2	3	4	5

Scoring: Add your scores in the following way:
1 Physically oriented = B + E + F + H + K + L + M
2 Psychologically oriented = A + C + D + G + I + J + N

monly used here and audio tapes are available demonstrating this technique. If your scores vary little between physical and mental approaches, you might benefit from either and this can only be determined by trying out some of both approaches.

Hardiness to stress

People react to stressful situations (stressors) in different ways. Some thrive, some suffer. Behavioural scientists have come up with a new concept to explain these discrepancies based on what they call 'hardiness'. Hardiness refers to an individual's ability to 'buffer' or moderate the effects of stress. It appears to consist of three interrelated factors—control, challenge and commitment—all of which reflect the ability to adapt to stressful situations.

Control refers to the perceived control a person has over his or her environment. It is known that those in high-stress jobs, for example police or ambulance officers, cope best while they feel in control of the situation.

Challenge refers to the degree to which a person sees a stressor as a challenge or a threat. If you regard a situation as a challenge, you're more likely to react to it positively than if you see it as a threat.

Commitment relates to the degree of meaning placed on a stressful event. If stressed people see their reaction to a stressor as meaningful for their future functioning, they place a greater commitment on mastering it.

In summary, stress appears to be an easy concept to understand—after all, we've all suffered from it at some stage. However, as can be seen from the simple outline above, there are many components that need to be taken into consideration in dealing with the problem. In the next chapter we look at a conceptual approach to coping with stress in general and some specific approaches to dealing with the milder, psychological stress outcomes in less 'hardy' individuals. Dealing with the more severe forms of stress and stress breakdown is a specialty area which is covered in other books.

Thought patterns and stress

In 1974, two sociologists, Stanley Cohen and Laurie Taylor, reported the results of years of work with prisoners who faced the prospect of spending their lifetimes locked away. They were interested in how these people survived mentally, even in the extreme conditions of solitary confinement. They looked at prisoners' thinking patterns and how their minds operated in order to survive, compared with those in the outside world.

To their amazement, they found that their thinking patterns—fantasies, day dreams, ideas of self—were no different from anyone else's. From this they concluded that we are all in a prison of sorts and that we all seek 'escapes' through the mind. Cohen and Taylor classified these mental 'escapes' using a number of different prison type analogies—'going over the wall', 'tunnelling under' etc. With no hope of physical escape, the prisoners used a variety of mental escapes—fantasy, imagination, dreaming, meditation, writing, creativity and even some strange hobbies. Prisoners serving life terms, even in solitary confinement, were able to create their own reality by THINKING their own reality.

Now this may sound strange, but logically it makes sense. We have a body which reacts to physical stressors and conditions. Animals are the same. In his book *Why Zebras Don't Get Ulcers*, Robert Sapolsky, a biologist from Stanford University, claims that we cope relatively well with the acute, or even chronic, stressors of being preyed upon, or having difficulty finding food in a drought. But animals don't worry themselves sick about these things. More to the point, they don't worry *in anticipation* that something bad may happen. Can you imagine if we humans had no mind, or absolutely no ability for thought associated with our body? We would react like an amoeba—withdraw wherever a stimulus threatened our physical being until that stimulus was removed, but never think about it!

We see something of this with reflex reactions. Place your hand on a burning stove and you immediately withdraw it, before you have time to think about it. As humans, we tend to think 'ouch, that hurt'. There's nothing wrong with this. It's very adaptive. But if we now begin to worry *in anticipation* that we will be burned if we're in the same room as a stove, that becomes stressful. It is the anticipation, which can only come from thought, which leads to the psychological stress which is characteristic of humans. As Mark Twain once said: '*My life has been full of catastrophes, most of which have never happened*'.

Looked at in this way, it's easy to see that stress is not so much what happens to you, but what you *think* about what happens to you and, more importantly, what *might conceivably* happen to you. If you *think* that you are in control of a situation, you're not likely to be stressed by that situation. If you *think* that someone is attacking your ego or integrity on the other hand, you're more likely to think other things such as 'I'm unworthy' or 'I'm useless'.

Let's be constructive. If thoughts *cause* stress, they can also help '*uncause*' it. The mind, after all, is under our control—although in most cases, we've let it run off on its own, thinking negative stress-arousing thoughts because these are easier, they get attention, it's a good way to cop out or merely because it requires effort to do otherwise. Irrespective of the cause, thought patterns can be changed. Just as an unfit body takes time and effort to get into condition, so does a wrong-thinking mind.

If we are to cope with the stress that can only come from the way we think, we must realise not just that something *can* be done, but that something *has* to be done with the way we think. We have pointed out the importance of escape—physical and mental—in helping 'empty' the mind of its negative, stressful thoughts and give us 'time out' to regroup. Now we need to look at ways of replacing those negative thoughts when they do occur, with other, more adaptive ones.

Re-programming the mind

You'll find no shortage of books, courses or lectures on ways of training the mind—'mind power', 'positive thinking', 'self-hypnosis', 'cognitive therapy'. You may have been turned off by their complexity. But many have something to offer.

We can think of the mind as a black box which, to all intents and purposes, can be 'emptied out'. Each thought arises like a minute spark in a fire which, if left uncontrolled, can flare into a blazing inferno. Most people's minds are blazing infernos of these uncontrolled thoughts all the time. And it's these that lead to stress. Hence, it's not only necessary to quell the flames, by 'escape', as we've already discussed, but to back-burn to regain control and manipulate thought patterns. This way, negative and largely irrational thoughts can be eliminated and positive thoughts put in their place.

Albert Ellis, an American psychologist, has developed a process to deal with this which he calls 'rational emotive therapy' or RET. The principle is simple and based on the acronym ABC. Ellis claims that stress is a consequence (C), of what we think is an adverse situation (A). In fact it's not—it's a consequence of a belief (B) about that adversity. For example, the adversity could be a difficult work situation, for which one individual has a belief that this is a threat (leading to stress), whereas another sees it as a challenge (leading to excitement). To change the consequences it's necessary to change the beliefs (B) about the adversity (A), rather than the adversity itself, which often can't be changed.

A (adversity) ⟶ usually leads to **C** (consequences)
but this ignores the intermediatory step
B (belief)
which must be changed to change the consequence
and this can be done by
D (disputing irrational beliefs)

Ellis claims that beliefs can be changed, although only through practice, by adding another letter to the formula—D for dispute. By actively disputing beliefs, we can change the way we think about stressors, and therefore ultimately reduce stress. Once you discover the belief associated with the stress, this is disputed by asking yourself a number of questions such as:

- Is there any evidence that this belief is actual reality?
- Where is this written down?
- What would happen if I didn't have this belief?
- What will happen if I continue to hold this belief?
- What could be the worst thing that can come of me not holding this belief?

As an example, let's take a work situation where a boss you don't get on with is an adversity (A) or stressor. The consequence (C) is anxiety, depression, anger—the gamut of typical reactions. But the boss may not be a stressor to fellow workers. Thus, it's your belief (B) about the situation—for example, I *must* impress this boss; I *must* be seen to do well; I *must* be successful, I *must not* let him wear me down—that is at the root of the stress. It's this *must*urbation, or demand for perfection, which Ellis claims is at the root of most disturbed thought. By challenging these thought patterns, as well as using techniques of mental and physical

---

GB high energy tip

Stop 'musturbating'. Irrationally thinking you *must* always achieve, win or be successful is one of the greatest causes of mental stress.

escape, it becomes possible to learn de-stressing techniques that can handle most day-to-day situations.

Albert Ellis has listed the 10 most common irrational beliefs (see box on p. 212) which lead to stress. He summarises these into three main categories:

1 The belief that I must always succeed;
2 The belief that you must be reasonable to me;
3 The belief that the world must treat me fairly.

Summary

As pointed out earlier, stress can range from being mildly annoying to severe, ultimately leading to breakdown or insanity. The techniques of stress management discussed here should not be seen as the solution to severe and chronic forms of stress, which may need the assistance of a health professional. The techniques also take time and practice to perfect. However, the stages of dealing with stress can be defined in most situations as:

1 recognise the problem and identify the source(s);
2 attempt to re-establish 'control';
3 practice an appropriate method(s) of escape;
4 re-program destructive thought patterns; to
5 turn maladaptive into adaptive stress; and
6 develop a personal 'hardiness' to stress.

Stress is something that will always be with us. Too little can lead to boredom and frustration; too much can be the kiss of death. The key to stress management is to find that optimal level of stress which enables you to be constructive and productive without interfering with your capacity for high level wellness.

Types of cognitive distortions or 'irrational thinking'

1 *All-or-nothing thinking* Seeing things in black and white, i.e. I'm a worthless person for being fat.

2 *Overgeneralisation* Where a single event is seen as a never-ending pattern of defeat, e.g. if I failed on that program, I'll fail on all programs.

3 *Mental filter* Where a single negative event is isolated and dwelt on to the isolation of all else, e.g. someone criticises you for being fat, so the world is a miserable place.

4 *Disqualifying the positive* Rejecting positive experiences on the basis that they 'don't count', e.g. losing some fat on fat measurements.

5 *Jumping to conclusions* Making a negative interpretation with facts:
   (a) *Mind reading*, i.e. concluding that someone is acting negatively to you.
   (b) *Fortune telling*, i.e. believing that things will turn out badly as a fact.

6 *Catastrophising* Seeing everything as a disaster, e.g. if I fail on this program, I might as well die.

7 *Emotional reasoning* Assuming your negative emotions reflect the way things really are, e.g. I think other people are looking at me, therefore it must be true.

8 *'Musturbating'* Using 'must' or 'should' statements, e.g. I 'must' not eat this cake or I will be a worthless person.
   (a) I 'must' succeed—or I'm a failure;
   (b) you 'must' treat me better—or you're a louse;
   (c) the world 'must' look after me—or it's a horrible place.

9 *Labelling* Applying a form of over-generalisation, e.g. I'm a loser for failing.

10 *Personalisation* Seeing bad things as being related just to yourself, e.g. only *I* don't have the will-power to keep exercising.

VII
Health screening

17 The risks that come with being fat, male and not a young buck any more

To this point we've looked at how to get fit and reduce fat. But, obviously, all of this could come to nought if you're stricken with one of the major ailments of the modern middle-aged man. Having high energy then, also means being free from disease and this is what this section is all about.

One of the most useful things about our 'modern' diseases is that they usually provide some kind of warning. Age, itself, is one of these. The marvels of medical science have yet to come up with a solution that reduces risks associated with the simple process of ageing. Hence, over the age of about 30 years, in men, things begin to break down. And, just as with your old car which you couldn't be bothered maintaining, a few squeaks and rattles suggest that something is likely to fall off very soon.

Being fat itself is another warning sign, or disease risk, for a range of different problems, not just fitting into tight spaces. Being fat around the middle (i.e. having a 'pot belly') is known to be an even bigger risk, for reasons which we've already outlined. Increasing age and increasing waist, are, therefore, the basis from which we begin this discussion of risk.

As well as the two risks mentioned above, the other main risks for men in middle age are:

- A history of any of the following in the family:
  — heart disease;
  — diabetes;
  — cancer;
  — high blood pressure;
  — high cholesterol.
- High blood pressure.
- High blood lipids (fats).
- High blood sugars.
- A high fat diet over many years.
- Smoking.

We'll look at each of these independently, but

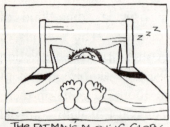

THE FAT MAN'S MORNING GLORY

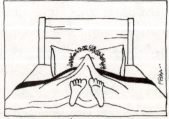

THE THIN MAN'S MORNING GLORY

briefly, before we go on to consider the diseases that they cause in the following chapter.

Family history

As one old University medical professor used to say: 'There's just two types of people. Those with good genes who don't need help, and those with bad genes who are beyond help.' Fortunately, it's not quite that bad. But genetics does have quite a role to play in risks of ill-health. Perhaps the most significant indicator of disease risk is family history (and particularly immediate family). Early death of one or both parents can indicate a need for special care and regular screening of the risks leading to that problem. While poor family health doesn't guarantee a bumpy road for life, it sure can throw up some significant warning signs.

Smoking

As any young woman can tell you, smoking can, and does, keep extra fat at bay. There's probably two reasons for this. First, nicotine has the effect of raising metabolic rate, meaning that more energy is burned at rest. Second, the process of holding a cigarette and regularly putting it in the mouth can have a relaxing effect and reduce the urge to nervously place food in there instead. It's well known that smokers who quit (and do nothing to compensate for the changes in metabolism) can gain up to 3.5 kg in weight over 12 months. Continuing to smoke, therefore, is often a tempting option for men who have weight on their mind.

However, despite these apparent advantages, smoking has one major disadvantage: it can kill you—through a number of painful means including lung cancer and heart disease. Smoking also increases the risk of other cancers (throat, bowel, intestine) and metabolic disorders such as diabetes. And, if that's not enough, the apparent maintenance of low body weight achieved through smoking is partly illusory. Research has now shown that smokers actually have a higher waist-to-hip ratio than non-smokers, even though they may be of a lower weight. When they quit, even if they put on weight, their waist-to-hip ratio (an indication of health risk) is likely to decrease, hence improving their chances from a health perspective. Overall then, there's little positive to be said for the evil weed.

Inactivity

Although it's most likely that by now you'll be regularly moving, both in a planned and 'incidental' fashion, you may have had a long period of inactivity in your life. And, while the evidence on exercise and reduced illness risk is still not clear, there's little doubt that inactivity is associated with a number of ailments, particularly heart disease, but also some cancers (e.g. bowel).

Blood pressure

Blood pressure (also called hypertension) is a measure of the pressure of blood in the arteries. There must be some pressure, but when this becomes too high it can put pressure on the heart and cause heart problems. High blood pressure is also often an indicator of other health problems.

Blood pressure (bp) measures are expressed as, for example, 120/100 where the first figure is the *systolic* bp and the second the *diastolic* bp. Systolic bp is the pressure in the arteries when the heart pumps; diastolic bp is the pressure between pumps. This can be compared to pressure inside a hose if a pump is attached and pumps in spurts. Like a hose which can clog up with mud, the arteries can clog up with fat, thus reducing the size of the hole, or lumen, through which blood flows, causing *atherosclerosis*. The artery walls may also lose their elasticity with age, lack of exercise and smoking and not be as responsive to expansion and contraction, leading to the complaint known as *arteriosclerosis*.

In the past, blood pressure has been classed as being 'mild', 'moderate', 'severe' or 'very severe'. But these are now thought not to adequately represent the role of high blood pressure as an important risk factor in heart disease. Instead, the US 'National Committee on Detection, Evaluation and Treatment of High Blood Pressure' has developed a number of new stages for hypertension (Table 17.1). This enables your doctor to classify blood pressure at different levels—normal and high normal, and then 4 stages of hypertension. Stage 1 hypertension used to be called 'mild'. High normal is regarded as an intermediary zone—the risk is not serious, but has the potential for getting worse, partic-

**Table 17.1   Classification of blood pressure
                categories**

Condition	Systolic bp	Diastolic bp	What to do
Normal	Less than 130	Less than 85	Recheck in 2 years
High-Normal	130–139	85–89	Recheck in 1 year
Hypertension			
Stage 1	140–159	90–99	Confirm within 2 months
Stage 2	160–179	100–109	See doctor within month
Stage 3	180–209	110–119	See doctor within week
Stage 4	210+	120+	See doctor immediately

ularly if there is hypertension in the family. Risks
increase with increasing stages of hypertension.

For many people, particularly those in the high
normal range, lifestyle changes can have the desired
effect on blood pressure reduction. There is a proportion of the population, however, who will find it necessary to use medication. Normal blood pressures are
around 120/80 and, while this generally increases with
age, there is no real reason why it should.

Blood sugars

High blood sugars are one of the first signs of diabetes
and this occurs when insulin loses its capacity to deliver
glucose to the cells of the body. When this happens,
blood sugars build up but the cells themselves are
starved of energy. A blood sugar reading, as determined
by a glucometer, can give an indication of the level of
sugars in the blood. Normal readings are between
5–10 mm; high readings 10+ mm. Chronically low
blood sugars are rare, but can occur in some cases of

GB high energy tip

Have regular check-ups. For men over 40 years of age a full medical check-up is recommended every 5 years; over 50, at least every 2 years.

---

hypoglycemia. Ironically, this occurs more readily in someone who eats too much refined sugar such that the system can no longer handle this.

Blood sugar levels can and do fluctuate between meals and as a result of exercise. However, the speed of increase of blood sugar is no longer thought to be simply a function of the sugar content of foods. Scientists have now established a 'glycaemic index' which indicates the speed with which the carbohydrates in food are absorbed into the bloodstream. This shows that not all foods that were once thought to affect blood sugar immediately (as is important for diabetes) do so. To measure these effects in the blood, blood sugar levels need to be taken over an extended period of several hours.

Blood fats

Blood fats are most important as an indicator of potential health problems. However, there is controversy and changing views about which fats are the most important. Historically, the following has been the development of scientific thought:

1 Total cholesterol is the best measure of heart risk (1970s).
2 Different lipoprotein components of cholesterol (particularly HDL and LDL) need to be taken into account with total cholesterol (1980s).

3   Total cholesterol and HDL and triglycerides all need
    to be considered (1990s).
4   Levels of anti-oxidants (more than 600 compounds in
    foods) also need to be considered with the above
    (1990s+).

The best advice that can be given at the moment is that:

- At least total and HDL cholesterol should be measured (HDL is normally around 20 per cent of the
  total and the higher it is and the lower total cholesterol is the better). A standard cut-off point for
  total cholesterol is 5.5 mmol/L.
- Cholesterol measures should be taken on more than
  one occasion. Winter and summer measures can be
  different.
- Fasting triglyceride measures should also be taken
  with cholesterol. This should also be low (i.e. below
  2 mmol/L).

Testing yourself for risks

Table 17.2 is a simple screening test for the six major
ailments of middle-aged men (each covered in detail in
the next chapter). Check yourself by beginning in the
left-hand column and ticking your risks. If any of these
apply to you, proceed to column 2 and check for major
symptoms of each of the ailments listed in column 3.
Columns 4 and 5 provide suggestions for tests which
can be carried out both at home and by your doctor
and column 6 suggests organisations that you might
contact for further information.

table 17.2 Screening test

Tick the following which apply to you:	Tick any of the following if you suffer regularly from:	This could indicate:	Check with your doctor for the following tests:	Also, regularly monitor your own:	For more information:
Overweight Smoker Over 35 years of age High blood pressure	Fatigue Tingling in fingers/toes Coldness Chest pain or pain down arms Shortness of breath Dizziness on exertion	Heart or vascular problems	Blood fats Blood pressure ECG (if appropriate)	Blood pressure (with a blood pressure cuff from any chemist)	National Heart Foundation (state offices)
High blood sugar Generally inactive High fat diet over many years	Frequent thirst Frequent urination Excessive hunger Lack of healing of wounds Fatigue/weakness Blurred vision	Diabetes	Glucose tolerance test	Blood sugar (with 'Clinistix' from any chemist)	Diabetes Australia (state offices)
History in the family of: • heart disease • diabetes • high blood pressure • bowel cancer • prostate cancer • arthritis	Blood in stools Infrequent/irregular motions Recent change in bowel habits Feeling of fullness Abdominal pain Feeling of incomplete emptying	Bowel cancer	Colonoscopy	Bowel motions	Anti-Cancer/Cancer Council (state offices). Gut Foundation (Prince of Wales Hospital, Randwick)

Tick any of the following if you suffer regularly from:	This could indicate:	Check with your doctor for the following tests:	Also, regularly monitor your own:	For more information:
Pain in right upper abdomen Frequent nausea/pain after eating Intolerance to fatty foods Yellow look Swollen ankles/feet/hands	Gallstones	X-Ray Ultrasound	Tolerance to fats	Your local doctor
Pain/burning on urination Feeling that bladder not emptied Poor urinary stream Pain in back/between anus and scrotum Dribbling after urination Difficulty starting urination	Prostate problems	Prostate check Biopsy Blood test	Urination	Anti-Cancer/Cancer Council (state offices)
Pain in testes Unusual swelling Pain on palpation Pain in lower abdomen Swelling of testes	Testicular cancer	X-Ray Ultrasound	Testes pain	Your local doctor
Joint pain/reduced flexibility Stiffness of joints on rising Excessive fatigue Fever Lack of appetite/weight loss	Arthritis	X-Ray Blood test	Joint pain	Arthritis Foundation of Australia (state offices)

If you have one or more ticks, go to column 2

18 The seven major health concerns of barrel-bellied men

Matters of heart—vascular disease

'Vascular' means 'relating to the blood supply'. The two main problems resulting from this in men are heart attack and stroke—both serious and both potentially fatal. They can also be a social disaster at parties. Both are closely associated with a pot belly.

Heart disease and stroke (more properly called 'vascular disease') are still the major killers in Western societies, being responsible for around 40 per cent of all deaths. Heart disease is also by far the major killer of men aged 35 plus. However, heart disease and stroke are on the decline, largely because of the decrease in smoking rates and some improvements in blood fat levels and blood pressure. Increases in abdominal obesity, on the other hand, may just turn these figures around again in the future. In any case, it's not much comfort to know that, as a man, vascular disease will kill about one in two of us.

In simple terms, a heart 'attack' occurs when the arteries, or main blood pipelines of the body, either block up because there's too much gunk flowing through them, or fail to expand and contract as they used to with the ebb and flow of blood being pumped from the heart. This puts pressure back on the pump (heart) and if this is weak or unconditioned (just like any underused muscle), a failure of blood and nutrients can cause the tissue to die—and whammo, a heart 'attack'!

You can think of a stroke as a 'heart attack of the brain' (or, alternatively, of a heart attack as a 'stroke of the heart'). Again, the problem is blood supply, but this time it's supply to brain tissue rather than heart. If bits of this don't get blood and so die, you can lose the functions of that part of the brain (left- or right-side movement, speech, etc.), even though the heart may be all right and still be able to supply blood to keep the rest of your body functioning. Stroke and heart attack then are both generally caused by decreased blood flow (ischaemia) resulting from blocking of the arteries.

Blocking of the arteries

Where arteries become blocked, the term that's used to describe this is *atherosclerosis*, which means a decrease in the size of the lumen, or hole, through which blood is pumped through the arteries (Figure 18.1). The 'gunk' that causes the build-up on the inside of the arteries is generally thought to be different types of fats from foods (including, but not restricted to, cholesterol). When coronary arteries (those supplying the heart with blood) become blocked, this is doubly serious because, like an army without food, it can stop supplies getting to the front line—the heart.

Where arteries lose their elasticity and ability to expand and contract, the term that's used is *arteriosclerosis* (note the subtle medical difference to confuse you). This simply means that there's more pressure on the heart because each time it pumps, the channel through which it pumps doesn't 'give' to relieve the pressure. Arteriosclerosis is one of those things that happens with age. But it doesn't necessarily have to. We know, for example, that smoking, poor diet and inactivity can decrease the ability of the arteries to expand and contract. And there's also a genetic factor involved.

To understand the difference between these two, think about a nice expandable plastic hose. It can get bigger or smaller according to the amount of water

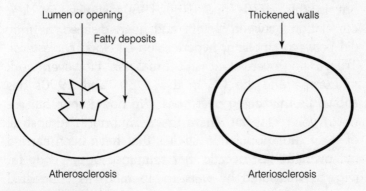

Lumen or opening

Fatty deposits

Thickened walls

Atherosclerosis

Arteriosclerosis

Figure 18.1

passing through it, but if there's also mud in the water this may eventually cling to the walls and clog up the hose, eventually blowing it off the tap—atherosclerosis. On the other hand, think of an old rubber hose. It doesn't expand and contract much, and even though there may not be much water coming through, if the water pressure is high enough it can still blow the hose off the tap—arteriosclerosis!

Now, having said all that, we'd have to say 'who cares'. If you're set for a heart attack you're not going to worry whether it's because the arteries are full of 'mud' or whether they're 'rubber' rather than 'plastic'. In either case, the solutions to the problem are the same. And one of the main solutions is—you guessed it—decreasing the middle tube.

A pot belly and heart attack

For a long time it was thought that being overweight was not a serious risk factor for heart disease and stroke. None of the major population studies carried out in the 1970s and early 1980s showed a clear correlation between weight and heart disease, as they did between smoking, hypertension or blood cholesterol. True. Being overweight isn't a real risk. However, work in Europe and the US in the 1980s and 1990s has shown us that being over*fat* is. We now know that it's not *if* you're fat but *where* that's important. Almost all of the major population studies that have been carried out over the last decade that examined upper body fat (e.g. as measured by waist-to-hip ratio) as contrasted with weight have shown a significant association between upper body fat—a pot belly—and vascular problems.

Of course, hindsight is a perfect science. It's now quite obvious why this would be so. The fat cells on the stomach of men (and post-menopausal women) are much more active in breaking down fat and pouring it into the bloodstream in response to demands for energy than fat cells elsewhere. This means that that fat (tummy fat), is much more likely to become the 'mud' in the hose that causes the heart or brain to die than fat which stays nice and snug in its little cellular homes whenever the pressure's on.

Imagine this: you've stored a few decent reserve picnics around the middle because times have been good, just like a bull in a paddock fattens up when the grass is green. Because you haven't had to do much to get to the land of milk and honey, the muscle that helps you to do active things (the heart) has also had a bit of a holiday. Now, all of a sudden, you get a bit stressed, or have to run to catch a bus. If this is extended, your muscles will call on the money you've saved in the belly to be paid back and used up as energy. Whoosh. Out it goes from fat cells into the bloodstream, filling up the arteries with mud and making it even harder for that poor little holidaying heart to get enough food to keep it alive. This is why pot belly equals vascular risk.

How do you know if it's coming on?

The most immediate symptom of a heart attack (in most cases) is a severe pain in the centre of the chest which may then radiate out to the inner arm or down the arms and legs. This can continue for minutes or hours giving a feeling of impending disaster and breathing difficulties. If this happens, get a doctor or ambulance immediately. In the meantime, if nothing else (such as a nitroglycerine tablet) is handy, have an aspirin and lie down.

Sometimes, impending symptoms of a heart attack can be signalled over quite a long period. Some patients complain of feelings of being cold, unusual fatigue, weakness, dizziness on exertion and a tingling feeling in the extremities (fingers or toes). Angina, which is a form of pain experienced as a result of ischaemia in the coronary vessels, is generally signalled by pains in the chest and arms on exertion. If you have the risk factors and these symptoms (listed in the health check on pages 223–4), you'd be well advised to consult you doctor as soon as possible.

What you can do yourself

After you've checked with your doctor, there are some things that you can do yourself to help monitor your situation, whether or not you have vascular problems.

1 *Blood pressure* Electronic blood pressure cuffs are so simple and cheap these days that you can teach your dog how to use them. There should be one in every home. However, if you're not scoring too well, don't panic. These machines aren't always as accurate as the manual ones. The first step would be to get an expert medical check.
2 *Blood fats* Blood fats such as cholesterol and triglycerides should be checked at least annually for men over the age of 35. Remember, they can also

be variable according to the time of the year and triglycerides vary according to whether you are fasted or not.

3 *Pulse checks* Regularly monitor your resting and exercise pulse for any irregularities or deviations from the normal. If there are big changes at any stage check with your doctor.

4 *Take regular aspirin* If you have any of the risk factors indicated in the health check on pages 223–4 and you have a history of heart disease in the family, a regular dose of half an aspirin per day *may* help prevent the problem *provided* that you are doing everything else in this program to help get rid of the fat. However, aspirin can cause bleeding from the lining of the stomach, so make sure your doctor knows you're taking it regularly.

Recognising heart attack symptoms

One of the big advances in heart disease detection in recent years has been the recognition of impending heart attack. Recognised warning signs now acknowledged are:

Chronic tiredness This is one of the least recognised but often persistent signs of trouble. Fatigue related to heart problems is generally regarded as abnormal.

Breathlessness This can occur during even mild exertion and results from the reduced blood flow resulting from even partial blockage of arteries. Inappropriate breathlessness should not be confused with normal breathlessness during exertion.

Pain Heart disease pain can radiate from the centre of the chest but be felt down the arms, in the jaw or across the shoulders. Exercise-related pain warning signs are back, pain or stomach pain or pressure. If these occur during exercise, you should stop and seek help. Heart attack pains are often confused with indigestion pains or even muscle soreness.

Feeling cold In some instances severe heart attack is preceded by smaller attacks which may go unnoticed. Feelings of cold, even in otherwise warm conditions, are a result of insufficient blood flow brought on by artery blockage.

Abnormal heart rhythm Arrhythmias, or abnormal heart rhythms (often felt as 'extra' or 'in between' beats), are quite common and often harmless. Arrhythmias during exercise, however, merit particular attention, especially if persistent.

Dizziness If this occurs after even mild exercise, it could be a result of reduced blood flow to the brain and could be a symptom of arterial blockage. Again, under these circumstances stop exercising and seek medical assistance.

Diabetes mellitus—the big belly problem

Diabetes means increased production of urine; *mellitus* comes from the latin word meaning honey. Hence diabetes mellitus is a syndrome (it's not a disease as such) where blood sugars flow over into the urine and are not used up in the cells as energy. There are two main types of diabetes:

1   Early onset, or that which occurs in young people largely as a function of a breakdown in the ability of the pancreas to produce insulin. This is genetically influenced. Because it requires regular insulin injections it's also called Insulin Dependent Diabetes Mellitus (IDDM).
2   Late onset, or that which occurs later in life (35+), is generally associated with overfatness. This often doesn't require insulin injections and hence is called Non-Insulin Dependent Diabetes Mellitus (NIDDM). It is this one that concerns us here.

Why a pot belly and (NIDDM) diabetes go together

Here is a very simple explanation of why 80–90 per cent of all late onset diabetes is associated with a pot belly.

Sugars from food, in the bloodstream, have to get into body cells to provide energy for life to proceed. They do this by being helped into the cell by the hormone insulin, which is secreted by the pancreas. Insulin acts as the gatekeeper to open the door for the sugars to get in. As body fat builds up around the belly, however, insulin becomes stressed to the maximum— like a doorkeeper trying to guard a bigger and bigger door—until it eventually gives up and walks out on the job, leaving all those sugar molecules banging on the door wanting to get in and party.

Why belly fat causes more angst for the insulin guards is not clear. It's probably because this has been the area developed in an evolutionary sense to store extra energy reserves in men and to give these up quickly. It's therefore likely to be the place where all the action is happening. In any case, we do know that the vast majority of the 3 per cent of the population who will develop late onset diabetes have a higher than recommended waist-to-hip ratio.

How do you know if you've got diabetes?

There are three main signs that might indicate a tendency towards diabetes and these should be taken especially seriously if you have carried a gut for a while, are now into your late thirties or early forties and if there is a history of diabetes or heart disease in the family. The signs are:

1   excessive urination (polyuria);
2   excessive hunger (polyphasia);
3   excessive thirst (polydypsea).

In addition, you may suffer periods of tiredness, weakness after effort, the need to get up often in the middle of the night to urinate and even some dizziness or eyesight failure. An even more telling sign (and often the clincher for some men) is that wounds seem to take forever to heal. If you have any of these symptoms, you might like to confirm it by testing your urine with some 'Clinistix' that can be purchased from any chemist. If this reads positive, go to the doctor for a glucose tolerance test as soon as possible.

Late onset diabetes does give some warnings, and if these are taken seriously (particularly by decreasing belly fat), the problem can sometimes be avoided. In the first instance there is a build up of blood sugars, which can be measured with a simple finger prick blood test or urine strip test. Second, there is a build up of insulin in the bloodstream (more complicated to measure) and, finally, there is full-blown diabetes. The medical warnings are summed up in a combination of measures known as 'syndrome X'. This includes high blood sugar, high blood pressure and high blood fats. If you are in any way suspicious of having diabetes or have the major risk factors (see pages 223–4), these three tests should be done regularly. See your doctor.

What you can do for yourself

It's estimated that about half of all diabetes is undiagnosed. In the 1960s it probably affected about 1 per cent of the population. But because diabetics now live to breed little diabetics, it's expected to increase to around 5 per cent of the population by the turn of the century. If you have any suspicions that you might have it (and a pot belly, high blood pressure and high cholesterol are a good indication), you'll need to be under medical supervision. After that you can:

1 *Check in with the Australian Diabetes Foundation* They'll provide all the information you need about managing your problem and also sell subsidised equipment such as blood sugar monitors etc.
2 *Monitor blood sugar* Use either a glucose strip or a blood glucose monitor (glucometer) obtainable from any chemist.
3 *Monitor blood pressure* Use an electronic blood pressure cuff purchasable from any chemist.

Keeping your eye on the bowl—colorectal cancer

Cancers of the colon and rectum (often called bowel

cancers) are the fastest growing form of cancer among men in Australia today. It's expected that it won't be long until these take over from lung cancer as the major form of cancer among men.

Cancers in the colon and rectum are literally a pain in the bum. But they don't necessarily show up that way. In fact, in many cases, the first sign of a problem shows up as blood in the stools—a good reason for keeping an eye on your outgoings as well as your incomings in any waist control program. By this time of course, a cancer can be well developed from the initially rather inoffensive polyps that usually precede it. Blood in stools must immediately be taken seriously—even if only a burst haemorrhoid is suspected.

Other symptoms of these types of cancer often depend on where the cancer is located. If it's in the left half of the large intestine it can tend to produce obstructive symptoms (e.g. constipation and a feeling of fullness) because the contents of the intestine here are relatively solid. There may also be a lot of gas and abdominal pain, or colic. Cancers of the rectum, being closer to the endpoint, usually produce symptoms earlier than colon cancers. Another common symptom here, together with bleeding, is a feeling of incomplete emptying of the bowel.

Right-sided colon cancers are much harder to detect because the intestinal contents here are much more fluid. This means that bleeding and mucous in the bowel motions are more hidden and not so easily noticed from a casual glance into the throne. Because they slowly bleed, however, they can lead to anaemia, or loss of iron in the blood, and this can lead to a feeling of continual tiredness.

Causes and cures

The causes of bowel cancer are not fully known; however, there is a high hereditary association. Anyone with a sibling or immediate parent with a detected cancer has an eight times greater risk of developing the cancer themselves and so should be on a regular screening regimen. What is known is that polyps that form in the intestinal tract seem to be precursors to cancer development, so ways of detecting and destroying these have now been developed through a technique called colonoscopy. This is where a flexible tube with a tiny video camera is passed into the rectum and into the colon—not the most pleasant of experiences, but certainly more pleasant than having the cancer.

Excess body fat, particularly in the form of a 'pot', has also been shown to have an association with these types of cancers, although it's not quite clear why. It may indeed not be the 'pot' itself, but what it's taken to get to this stage—a high fat diet. Even alcohol has been suspected. As with most cancers, smokers are also at increased risk. A high level of fibre in the diet, as is recommended in any good waist control program, can help reduce the incidence of the problem.

If a cancer is detected, it may be quite simply removed if it's caught early enough. The problem, of course, is that this may have spread, not only to other parts of the colon, in which case some of this may have to be removed, but to other organs, such as the liver and gall-bladder. If too large a section of the colon has to be removed, and if this is too close to the rectum for it to be rejoined, the end of the bowel may need to be brought to the skin surface. In this case waste contents then have to be kept in a bag, called a colostomy bag. These days, this is the exception rather than the rule.

What you can do for yourself

Apart from regular check-ups after the age of 40 (particularly if there is a history of bowel cancer in the family) the most important things a man can do to protect against the disease are:

- *Keep your eye on the bowl* At the first sign of blood in your motions, see your doctor.
- *Be aware of changes in bowel habits* Any significant changes—increased constipation or increased diarrhoea—should be monitored closely.

How not to be prostrate with prostate cancer

If cancer of the bowel is a pain in the bum, cancer of the prostate is a pain near the bum—more accurately between the anus and scrotum. It can also manifest as pain in the lower back, and this can sometimes be confused with back problems.

The prostate is a small gland, situated at the base of the bladder. Its function is the injection of seminal fluid into the urethra which enables sperm to be produced from the penis on ejaculation. There are a number of things that can happen to the prostate, but perhaps the most significant, because it's potentially fatal, is a cancerous growth. This is not to say that all growths of the prostate are cancerous. In fact, around 50 per cent of middle-aged men have what is commonly called 'benign hypertrophic prostate', or enlargement of the prostate which is not cancerous. This can cause some symptoms, such as lower back ache. But, in the benign case, the tumour is not expanding, and hence presents no danger to other organs.

The most significant symptoms of prostate problems are:

- difficulty in urinating;
- a feeling of fullness, even on emptying the bladder;
- pain on urination;
- lower back pain;
- pain between the scrotum and anus.

There is not a lot of strong evidence on the association of abdominal fatness with prostate problems. But then there's not a lot of knowledge about any of the causes of prostate cancer. We do know that there is a strong familial tendency such that prostate cancers, like many other cancers, can run in families. There's also a likelihood that, as with other cancers, abdominal fat, and the problems that go with it, are not likely to reduce your risks. Age is the other predominant risk factor. And, like the other illnesses examined here, age and a 'pot belly' go together like hand in glove.

Speaking of hand in glove—diagnosis of prostate problems, like other problems that occur inside downstairs, is not always a pleasant experience. It involves a gloved finger being inserted into the anus by a doctor with a skilled touch. If an enlarged prostate is detected, other tests then need to be carried out to confirm whether this is cancerous or benign.

Treatment can be very effective if the problem is caught early enough. And while this may cause infertility, it rarely leads to impotence. If such is the patient's desire, a healthy sex life can be maintained after prostatectomy. Although not as common as other forms of cancer, such as lung and bowel cancer, prostate disease is growing in importance in men. It's well worth having an annual check up after about the age of 50, and particularly if there are problems in the family.

What can you do for yourself?

The answer in this case is very little. Waterworks problems should be observed very closely and any changes in usual patterns, such as decreased flow of urination, pain on urination, feelings of fullness etc., that cannot be associated with lifestyle changes should be checked immediately.

Fat, flatulent, fair and forty plus

Gallstones are a typically Western fat disorder. They are almost unheard of in native populations with low-fat and high-fibre diets, yet the common indicators in Western cultures have for years been described as:

- fair
- fat
- female
- flatulent
- fiftyish

Gallstones are almost twice as common among over-weight females as males. But the incidence is increasing in males. And while they are unlikely to be fatal, they can be a real damn nuisance, and quite painful to boot.

What are gallstones?

The gall-bladder is a small organ attached to the liver. Its function is to produce bile acids for the digestion of fat. When fat is eaten in the diet, the gall-bladder squirts bile into the stomach to help break it down to its component parts for distribution around the body.

The trouble is that bile acids actually come from cholesterol, which is manufactured in the liver, as well as coming from food sources—generally saturated fat in the diet. Too much cholesterol can lead to an overloading of the gall-bladder and the formation of crystals, which are literally like little stones throughout the gall-bladder.

The main symptoms of gallstones are:

- pain in the upper right abdominal cavity;
- an intolerance to fatty foods;
- flatulence;
- reddenning of the palms and swollen joints in some cases.

Gallstones in men are typically a 'pot belly' problem. It's the extra mobile fat circulating in the system from abdominal fat cells that just overloads the gall-bladder until such time as it decides to 'pack up'. The best method of attack, then, is prevention. Don't develop the porch over the playpen in the first place. Or if you've got one, get rid of it. You can live without a gall-bladder, but most things were put there for a purpose and you're better off hanging on to what you've got if you can.

Treatment

The treatment for gallstones has traditionally been removal of the gall-bladder. However, with new technology stones can be shattered with laser beams, or extracted through a tiny incision using a laproscope. Again, these techniques are never always guaranteed, so it's best not to wait for it to happen.

If the gall-bladder is removed, the bile duct, which joins the gall-bladder to the liver, is used as the source of bile for digesting fats. The size of this, though, restricts its effectiveness and could be one way, if nothing else works, to get you to decrease fatty foods in the diet. It is a harsh form of treatment though.

Testicular cancer: the growing male problem

Testicular cancer has been called the male equivalent of breast cancer. And while cancer of the testes doesn't yet kill as many men as breast cancer kills women, it is rapidly becoming a major health concern. Currently it's the most common cancer in men aged between 20 and 35. Prostate cancer and testicular cancer together account for as many deaths annually as breast cancer in women.

Symptoms of testicular cancer are lumps, changes in size of the testes, and heaviness and pain in the scrotal region or lower abdomen. If detected early, the prognosis is positive, with 95 per cent of men surviving more than 5 years after detection.

What can you do for yourself?

Like breast cancer, testicular cancer can also be detected early by self-examination. Yet, unlike breast cancer self-examination, which is familiar to over 90 per cent of women, testicular self-examination is virtually unknown among men.

In a recent survey of over 16 000 European male students, English researchers found that over 87 per cent had never examined themselves for testicular irregularities (the first sign of carcinoma). Only 3 per cent claimed to regularly examine themselves.

Men interviewed also regarded testicular cancer as of much less concern than breast cancer in women, even though women who were interviewed rated the male form as serious a concern for men as breast cancer in women. Clearly, there is a deficiency in understanding and education relating to men's health problems in contrast to women.

Testicular self-examination (TSE) involves mild palpitation of the testes to feel for soreness or irregularities. These should be immediately reported to a doctor for further examination. Failure of early detection can mean a significant increase in the risk of death, and hence all possible irregularities should be reported.

An old friend—Arthur Itis

Arthritis is one of the most common symptoms associated with ageing. It's so common, in fact, that there are reports that there has never been a skeleton examined over 70 years of age that doesn't show some signs of it. It seems like we'll all get it somewhere—if we hang around long enough. Where, how bad, and what type, seems to be as much based on the luck of the draw as anything although, as with most of these problems, it's always helpful to be able to choose your parents wisely.

There have been suggestions that joint damage through excessive regular physical activity early in life may be a cause of arthritis later. But research recently carried out on the older bodies of former athletes in Sweden suggests that, if anything, regular exercise decreases the risk of arthritis. Severe trauma to joints from contact sports such as football and boxing and motor vehicle injuries early in life, however, may have an impact and may lead to later joint dysfunction, but even this is not clear.

Because heredity appears to play a part, anyone with problems in the family needs to take care. Diet might also be important and it's more than likely that what diet and a lack of exercise do (i.e. make you fat), is the big unknown factor in arthritis. The pressure on weight bearing joints such as the knees, ankles and hips, is obviously greater with excess body weight. And because most men put this excess on around the middle, there is a fair correlation of belly size with arthritis severity. With women, it's known that any increases in obesity can cause an increased risk of arthritis.

Even slight reductions of body fat can help to give the arthritis patient some relief. Careful attention to diet can help add to this.

What is arthritis?

Arthritis is pain caused by the mechanical wearing away, or inflammation, of bone joints. In the overweight, as we've seen, it's most common in the big joints of the knees and ankles, but it can also strike the fingers and toes. There are two main forms. Osteo-arthritis is caused by the 'wearing away' of the bones at the joints ('osteo' = bone). Bone cells generally readily regrow. But in this type of arthritis, the matrix of bone, which is a bit like a cement column holding up a building, tends to thin out and wear away.

Rheumatoid arthritis arises from inflammation of the tissue around the joints and can occur more frequently in the back and neck. This is likely to be more painful, more consistent and probably even harder to deal with than osteo-arthritis, but is probably less related to early trauma.

Things that won't help arthritis

There are many 'quack' remedies on the market to reduce the pain from arthritis. Most of them have no supportive scientific evidence, but it should be said that some do work for some people. Whether this is psychological or not is probably not important provided that the treatment involved is not dangerous or likely to interfere with your wallet. In any case, if any of these are used, they should be combined with, and made secondary to, a reduction in body fat. This is going to be the big one in the long run.

Other treatments that are about include copper bracelets, gold injections, restriction of certain foods and acupuncture. Arthritics often claim to also have a built-in weather forecasting ability. The old saying is '. . . *aches and pains, storms and rains*', and while many doctors have rubbished this over the years, recent research from the US has shown that it may not be so crazy after all.

The mechanisms by which this happens are not clear. However, it's quite possible that changes in barometric pressure can be sensed in the joints without being sensed perceptively. After all, this is explained as the mechanism behind migrating birds and changes in animal behaviour patterns. So why could it not happen to humans—even fat ones?

What can you do for yourself?

Again, the answer to this is unclear. Reducing body fat and maintaining fitness will certainly help. Regular use of the joints can also help maintain their integrity. If weight-bearing exercise for this is painful, hydrotherapy, or exercises in warm water, may be the answer. Some people also find avoiding meat helps the problem, but there are wide individual differences in this.

Like most health problems, the best solution is obviously not to have the problem in the first place. For someone with a genetic tendency towards arthritis, care of body weight, diet and a regular program of full range-of-motion exercise is likely to help. But even then, as with most things, there is no real guarantee.

Index